HEALING SPICES

HEALING
SPICES

50 WONDERFUL SPICES, AND HOW TO USE THEM
IN HEALTH-GIVING FOODS AND DRINKS

KIRSTEN HARTVIG

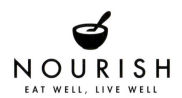

NOURISH
EAT WELL, LIVE WELL

Dedicated to Bob

Healing Spices
Kirsten Hartvig

First published in the UK and USA in 2016 by
Nourish, an imprint of Watkins Media Limited
19 Cecil Court
London WC2N 4EZ

enquiries@nourishbooks.com

Managing Editor: Rebecca Woods
Editors: Carolyn Ryden, Elinor Brett
Designers: Jade Wheaton, Suzanne Tuhrim

A CIP record for this book is available from the British Library

ISBN: 9781848991545

1 3 5 7 9 10 8 6 4 2

Typeset in Futura
Colour reproduction by XY Digital
Printed in China

PLEASE NOTE
The nutritional and calorie information is based upon the ingredients listed for each recipe, not for any alternative ingredients or additional serving suggestions.

MEASUREMENTS
Do not mix metric and imperial measurements.
1 tsp = 5ml   1 tbsp = 15ml   1 cup = 240ml

DISCLAIMER
The information in this book is intended to be helpful and informative. It is not meant to replace professional medical advice, and should be used at the reader's discretion. While every care has been taken in compiling the recipes for this book, Watkins Media Limited, or any other persons who have been involved in working on this publication, cannot accept responsibility for any errors or omissions, inadvertent or not, that may be found in the recipes or text, nor for any problems that may arise as a result of preparing one of these recipes.
If you are pregnant or breastfeeding or have any special dietary requirements or medical conditions, it is advisable to consult a medical professional before following any of the recipes contained in this book. Some foraged ingredients such as berries can be fatally poisonous. Neither the publisher nor the authors can take any responsibility for any illness or other unintended consequences resulting from following any of the advice or suggestions in this book.

CONTENTS

INTRODUCTION

I have often wondered why nations fought such long wars over nutmeg, cloves, vanilla and black pepper. It seems disproportionate to have risked lives just for an added flavour. Had it been food wars, not spice wars, it would be easier to understand. However, spices are much more than wonderful taste supplements. They also provide concentrated, powerful medicines that can enhance health and vitality, treasures that ancient cultures knew well and that modern society is now rediscovering through science and research.

ABOUT THIS BOOK

The spices described within this book come from all over the world. Many are related and belong to the same genus or botanical family – for example, chillies and paprika; ginger, galangal, turmeric and zedoary; and all the peppercorns. Most originate from tropical equatorial regions and dry mountainous areas, though there are some notable exceptions such as salt, which is a mineral that comes (essentially) from the sea, and juniper, which is common throughout the Northern Hemisphere.

As you read the spice profiles that follow, you will discover the history, geography and science of the ingredients stored in your spice cupboard, and learn where to buy them, how to store them and how best to utilize them as both flavourings and medicines. I also hope to introduce you to spices that you may not have encountered before: perhaps melegueta pepper, kaffir lime leaves or sansho?

With a choice of nearly 100 recipes from around the world as well as in-depth profiles of 50 key spices, you will learn how to create a whole range of dishes, preserves, spice blends, beverages and cordials. All the spices that I feature are available either in supermarkets, health food stores, Asian supermarkets or from online suppliers. Some, such as turmeric and galangal, are also becoming much easier to find fresh as interest in exotic ingredients has increased their demand. The ingredients I have chosen in my recipes are not expensive, although I always encourage the use of organic ingredients and locally sourced, seasonal produce. As the world shrinks and multiculturalism takes root, our food choices grow more interesting, allowing us to explore other cuisines and dare to experiment to make them our own.

In writing *Healing Spices*, my aim has been to produce a complete, easy-to-use, practical guide to the flavoursome world of spices, and to tell you all that you need to know in order to release their potential for improving your wellbeing. The spices that I include have had a worldwide impact on traditional and contemporary cooking, and each (used correctly) has the ability to transform a dish from the ordinary to the extraordinary. Some of my choices, such as garlic, horseradish and cocoa, are not spices by definition, but they are included here as significant members of an expanding palette of ingredients essential to bring out the flavour and give identity to today's international cuisines.

In a world that is awash with taste-alike processed foods and synthetic flavourings, I hope that this book will inspire you to experiment with, and extend, your spice range, and to deepen your understanding of the wisdom of cultures for whom the use of spices has long been an essential part of the fabric of daily life.

ABOUT SPICES

Spices are the aromatic, fresh or (more commonly) dried barks, roots, berries, buds, fruits, leaves, grains and seeds of a variety of trees, shrubs and plants, and have been treasured for their healing and taste-enhancing effects since the earliest times. The ability of spices to transform bland foods to attractive meals and medicines is well illustrated in traditional cuisines all over the world.

Cloves from the Moluccas; cinnamon from Sri Lanka; pepper from the Malabar Coast; chillies from Peru: for over 4,000 years, spices from five continents have been used to bring recipes to life, to enhance beauty and vitality, and to treat and prevent diseases. They have enriched our language and our folklore, excited our senses and inspired us to explore new culinary vistas.

Spices have also played a central role in the development of world trade – in our long search for them we have discovered new lands, fought fierce wars, earned and lost fortunes, and changed political destinies. Today, nearly 2 million tonnes of spices are grown, processed, traded and sold each year around the world.

The word 'spice' comes from the French *épice*, which itself derives from the Latin word *species*, meaning type, specific kind or ware. Most dictionaries define a spice as something aromatic or pungent, used alone or in combination with other ingredients to flavour food, but it also means something that adds interest and excitement. Spices are mostly dried, concentrated substances, used primarily for seasoning and are best added at the beginning of the cooking process as heat brings out the richness of their full flavours.

In cooler parts of the world, salt is the most common indigenous spice, used for centuries to give or improve flavour, and to preserve and cleanse. In hotter regions, and especially in the tropical regions that lie either side of the equator, the sun has more power, plants grow faster, flavours are stronger and food goes off more quickly, so the need for effective preservatives and disinfectants is greater. Perhaps this, in part, explains the fact that most of the spices we value so highly today (cinnamon, pepper, ginger, vanilla, nutmeg, cloves and chillies) are native to the tropics of Asia, Central America and Africa.

In a multicultural world where what was once considered foreign and exotic has become commonplace, it is easy to forget that most spices come from plants native to very particular local environments and were once completely unknown outside these areas. A small group of remote tropical islands (the Moluccas, or Maluku, in Indonesia) was the birthplace of nutmeg and cloves, once the world's most treasured spices, and the Mediterranean provided a suitable cradle for many of the aromatic spices now popular worldwide, such as cumin and coriander, fennel and fenugreek, poppy, nigella and aniseed.

As the pace of world trade and population migration increased, the Americas and the Caribbean islands became melting pots for many disparate cooking traditions, mixing the indigenous Aztec and Inca cuisines with those of European

THE ORIGIN OF SPICES WITHIN THIS BOOK

INDIA/HIMALAYAS/SRI LANKA

ajowan	cardamom	ginger	lemongrass
amchoor	cinnamon	jaggery	pepper
black cumin	curry leaf	kokum	zedoary

AMERICAS/CARIBBEAN

allspice	cocoa	pink pepper
chilli	paprika	vanilla

MEDITERRANEAN/MIDDLE EAST

aniseed	cumin	horseradish	poppy seed
celery seed	fennel seed	mahlab	saffron
coriander	fenugreek seed	pomegranate seed	

ASIA

asafoetida	caraway	kaffir lime leaves	turmeric
bay leaf	garlic	nigella	

CHINA

cassia	galangal	star anise	Szechuan pepper

SPICE ISLANDS

cloves	nutmeg	mace

AFRICA

melegueta pepper	tamarind

JAPAN

sansho	wasabi

EUROPE

juniper	mustard

conquerors and African slaves. Spices from Asia were planted in New World colonies and New World spices were introduced to countries in the Mediterranean and the Far East.

Spices are now cultivated in many more parts of the world, particularly in Asia. Individually and in mixtures, they are an essential and valuable part of the Earth's nourishing and healing ability: creating balance, giving strength and enhancing the health and immunity of the world's inhabitants.

THE SPICE TRADE

The story of the ancient spice trade is full of mystery and romance. Spices were transported around the globe by boat, and in the quest to find new, faster routes and more valuable spices, continents and islands were discovered by chance. It was in his attempt to find a shortcut to the Indian Ocean and Asia, for example, that Christopher Columbus accidentally landed on an island off the coast of Central America (hence the confusing name of the West Indies being given to islands in the Caribbean). Although Columbus failed to find Asia, he discovered amazing riches

PERCENTAGE OF
WORLD SPICE TRADE
ORIGINATING FROM
THE NINE AREAS

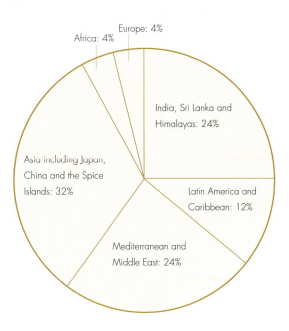

Europe: 4%

Africa: 4%

India, Sri Lanka and Himalayas: 24%

Asia including Japan, China and the Spice Islands: 32%

Latin America and Caribbean: 12%

Mediterranean and Middle East: 24%

in the form of hitherto unknown foods and spices, including tomatoes, potatoes, quinine, corn, cocoa, allspice, chillies and vanilla, which quickly became highly valued commodities.

The oldest records of spices being traded come from Egypt, about 3,500 years ago, where a relief sculpture in a burial monument by the Nile shows a series of canals and lakes linking the river with the Red Sea. Ancient Egyptians took this route to reach Africa and India via the Arabian Sea in search of pepper, cinnamon and other Asian condiments. There were also overland trade routes, and as far back as 2000 BC the Phoenicians are known to have traded spices along the Mediterranean coast from Lebanon (and even reached as far north as Cornwall, according to some, and to Africa and India). Ancient Greeks and Romans flavoured and preserved their food with spices and utilized the Silk Route to China to trade spices, too.

As the centuries unrolled and power shifted, the Moors came to dominate the Mediterranean trade and took local spices over to Asia, where the taste for them grew. At the same time, Chinese traders sold cassia and star anise, and visited the Moluccas (later known as the Spice Islands and now, the Maluku) in the South China Sea to source cloves, nutmegs and mace. Ships on the trade routes passed the Malabar Coast to pick up peppercorns, and Venetian traders also started sending ships to collect spices from along the North African coast to take north into Europe. As a result, Venice became increasingly powerful, prosperous and beautiful, and the envy of the rest of Europe.

From the earliest times, traders had a habit of keeping the origins of their spices secret in order to control their market, and often charged outrageous prices for their much-in-demand cargoes. Fortunes were made and lost as nations competed to find and distribute the spices from Asia as speedily as possible, and new routes were constantly sought. The Portuguese found the passage around South Africa's Cape of Good Hope to the Indian Ocean and the South China Sea, which brought them new wealth and power, but Spain was in the game, too, with Columbus's Atlantic adventures unlocking the aromatic riches of the Caribbean Islands and Central and South America.

The Portuguese and the Spanish adventurers were followed by the British and the Dutch, who set up the mighty East India Companies and spent years fighting over the Spice Islands and other important Asian spice havens. They guarded their territories fiercely and created spice monopolies, which were only broken when Pierre Poivre (known to the English-speaking world as Peter Piper) established a new pepper plantation on the island of Mauritius with seeds and cuttings he had stolen from the Spice Islands.

Sadly, the raging Spice Wars of the 17th century, and the many conflicts and skirmishes that preceded and followed them in the pursuit of wealth and dominance, had even darker consequences for countless thousands of indigenous peoples who were brutally robbed of their lands and livelihoods by European greed. Peaceful, often highly evolved societies were colonized and destroyed within decades of the Europeans' arrival, and the ruthless desire of the spice traders for power and money fuelled the 350-year obscenity known as the North Atlantic slave trade.

Meanwhile, the spices survived and thrived in their native habitats and became highly valued commodities overseas. They are now established and cultivated in many other parts of the world with suitable climates and growing conditions. Today, the nations of the Western world have become the world's largest spice consumers.

SPICES AS FOOD

As more people seek to live more healthily, the global market that the spice trade helped to create offers us a wealth of opportunity to improve the nutritional quality of our diets. The near-magical ability of spices to transform simple foods into memorable feasts can help us to rebalance our diet in satisfying ways, and their powerful health-protecting and immune-stimulating properties can help us to deal more effectively with the stresses of modern living.

Spices enhance the five essential tastes: sweet, salt, sour, bitter and hot, and equally importantly, they preserve freshness, add colour and aid digestion. The key to effective cooking with spices is to remember that they should always enhance the flavours and qualities of the other ingredients, and never overpower them. Celebrating the quality of raw materials should be the aim, and no one flavour should upset the balance of a dish as a whole taste experience.

Spicy foods are not everyone's choice, of course, and some people have a particular aversion to 'hot' flavours. Children, for example, have extremely sensitive palates and generally prefer sweetly aromatic spices such as vanilla, cinnamon and star anise to the pungency of ginger, chilli and garlic. This should not deter you from using spices in family dinners: most people, young and old, enjoy sausages, which would not taste nearly so good without their added spices. Just go easy on the hotter ingredients when preparing main dishes, and make some hot and spicy condiment mixtures for those who have stronger palates to help themselves to at the table.

When possible, buy spices whole and grind them only as needed, either with a pestle and mortar or a coffee grinder. Store them in airtight containers and keep out of direct sunlight. Some, such as nutmeg, will keep for many years, but it is better to buy most spices in small amounts and replace them annually. One of my friends buys herself new spices every year as a birthday present, and her fabulous cooking is much enhanced as a result. The same storage rule also applies to dried herbs, which are often placed alongside spices in the kitchen. In broad terms, herbs are greener, gentler and less pungent, and better suited to being added at the end of the cooking process.

Heat brings out the full flavour and aroma of most spice seeds, so they are often toasted on their own in a hot pan before any oil or other ingredients are added. Be vigilant as it is all too easy to burn them at this stage. Other spices release their flavour when dissolved in hot water, and others are best introduced just before serving to ensure perfect seasoning. Salt and pepper are often added this way, as are jaggery and wasabi.

Eating a balanced and varied diet pepped up with tastes redolent of far-flung places adds real spice to life. If you learn about the environments in which individual spices thrive and are able to reproduce the right conditions at home, you can probably grow your own spice plants too. Sunny borders and yards, greenhouses, south-facing balconies and windowsills, and vertical gardens created in urban windows can provide the perfect environment for growing spices such as caraway, mustard, poppies, saffron, horseradish and chilli; and the pride and joy of picking your own fresh flavourings at home is priceless. Just remember that spices thrive on careful nurture in terms of watering, weeding and pest control.

SPICES AS MEDICINE

The ancient Greek physician Hippocrates famously advised: 'Let food be thy medicine and thy medicine be thy food', and including spices in our diet should help us to approach this ideal. Not only have spices helped shape the economic structures of the modern world, but they have also helped to underpin the development of human civilization.

For thousands of years before the development of modern medicine, spices were valued for their ability to help people resist disease and maintain good health, although their essential nutrients, antioxidants and health-enhancing phytochemicals had not been isolated and identified. The ancient civilizations of Mesopotamia,

Egypt, China and India prescribed spices in a wide range of medicines to treat infections and infestations, relieve pain, cleanse wounds, ease digestion, aid sleep and purify the air. By understanding the importance of spices in traditional medicine, we can perhaps approach an understanding of how ancient cultures managed not only to thrive, but also to reach extraordinary levels of sophistication. Centuries ago, people lived without computers and laboratory experiments, but they knew how to turn the pods of the vanilla orchid into a fragrant spice, how cloves could relieve toothache, and that poppy seed heads made a sedative tisane. They knew that spices made food easier to digest, less prone to go off and more bug proof. They also knew how spices could transform a simple dish into something extraordinary, helping food to become medicine, literally.

It is not surprising, therefore, that modern science confirms the nutritional value and medicinal properties of a wide range of spices, nor that the pharmaceutical industry is discovering increasing numbers of possible applications for spice-derived chemicals in the treatment of contemporary illnesses, including cancer and viral infections. At home, minor ailments can often be treated successfully with spices, either as part of a meal, or in a tea, poultice or gargle (or even simply washed down with a glass of water).

These days, most spices are consumed far from where they are grown, and many are cultivated far from their original habitats. Some are used dried, others fresh, but all are highly potent and make a valuable addition to the kitchen spice rack and the natural medicine cabinet. Recognized as powerful disinfectants, medicines and food preservatives, spices are part of the wonder of nature, as we are part of nature and it is part of us. If we can live with respect for the bounty to be found in our natural environment, it can play an important role in helping us to find health and happiness.

THE SPICES

This chapter will introduce you to the world of spices, explaining the history and culinary and medicinal uses of nearly 50 major spices. Ten spices stand out as 'Super Spices' and are highlighted with gold introductory text (and in capitals below). They were once extremely valuable (some were, literally, worth their weight in gold) and have long been treasured for their effects on food and health. Now all kinds of spices are attracting huge interest from the pharmaceutical industry because of their many medicinal properties and the potential they might have in the prevention and treatment of many of the most serious diseases of our time.

Ajowan	Curry Leaf	NUTMEG
Allspice	Fennel Seed	Paprika
Amchoor	Fenugreek Seed	PEPPERCORNS
Aniseed	Galangal	Pink Peppercorns
Asafoetida	Garlic	Pomegranate Seed
Bay Leaf	Ginger	Poppy Seed
Black Cumin	Horseradish	Saffron
Caraway Seeds	Jaggery	Salt
Cardamom	Juniper	Sansho
Cassia	Kaffir Lime	STAR ANISE
Celery Seed	Kokum	Szechuan Pepper
CHILLI PEPPERS	Lemongrass	Tamarind
CINNAMON	Mace	TURMERIC
CLOVES	Mahlab	VANILLA
Cocoa	Melegueta Pepper	Wasabi
Coriander	MUSTARD SEED	Zedoary
Cumin	NIGELLA SEEDS	

Ajowan *Trachyspermum ammi*

Native to India, Pakistan, Iran and Afghanistan, ajowan is a member of the parsley family (*Apiaceae*) is also known as ajwain seed, carom, *vaamu*, *omam*, ajowan caraway and bishop's weed. It is extremely popular in southern Indian-style cooking, and is used also in many North African spice mixtures, including Berbere (see page 108). The flavour is reminiscent of thyme due to the presence of the essential oil thymol, and in Indian cooking the seeds are added to bean dishes, breads, cookies and savoury pastries. This may be because ajowan seeds are thought to relieve indigestion and wind. Ajowan closely resembles lovage seed in appearance and, confusingly, is sometimes referred to as such in Indian recipes.

BUYING AND STORING

Ajowan is available as whole seeds from Asian food stores and the fresher the seeds, the stronger their flavour. The seeds can be stored for up to 2 years in an airtight container kept out of direct sunlight.

FOOD PROFILE

Ajowan seeds, which in botanical terms are actually fruit pods, have an aromatic, pungent and slightly bitter taste that lies somewhere between thyme and aniseed, and they should be used sparingly to avoid overpowering other flavours in a dish. When chewed, they have an intensely hot, tongue-numbing effect. Once crushed, the seeds release a strong smell of thyme. They go well with all starchy foods, such as root vegetables, breads, grains and pulses, and add a distinctive savoury flavour to chutneys, pickles and relishes. Roasted ajowan seeds can also be used sprinkled on vegetables and salads, or added to stews, stir-fries and casseroles.

NUTRITIONAL PROFILE

The seeds have a sharp, strong thyme flavour due to their essential oil content, which is over 50% thymol, a strong antiseptic, antibiotic and antifungal. The essential oil also contains limonene, terpinene, cymene and carvacrol.

HEALTH PROFILE

In India, dried ajowan seeds are powdered and soaked in milk, which is then filtered and given to babies and young children to treat colic and stomach ache. For adults, a spoonful of seeds crushed with a pinch of salt and taken with a glass of water is said to relieve stomach pain and indigestion. 'Omam water' is a tisane of ajowan seeds infused in hot water, which is taken to treat colds, cough, headaches, heartburn, allergies and arthritic pain.

The main active ingredients in ajowan are thymol and acetylcholine. Thymol is a strong antiseptic, popular in toothpastes and mouthwashes; acetylcholine has a relaxing effect on the digestion and the circulation.

NOTE:

- Lovage seeds and dried thyme can be used as culinary substitutes for ajowan in many recipes.

Allspice *Pimenta dioica*

A member of the myrtle family (*Myrtaceae*), allspice is also known as myrtle pepper, pimenta, pimento, newspice and Jamaica pepper. The explorer Christopher Columbus first came across the spice on the island of Jamaica in the Caribbean when on one of his voyages west to the New World. He introduced it to Europe in the belief that it was pepper, hence its appellation *pimenta*. It was later given the name 'allspice' by English spice merchants who thought it tasted like a combination of cinnamon, nutmeg and cloves, with a hint of peppery mace.

Allspice is made from the dried berries of an evergreen tree native to the West Indies and Central and South America. For centuries it was thought that the plant would grow only in Jamaica because trees planted elsewhere rarely thrived. The allspice plant is frost tender but can be grown indoors as a houseplant, or in a greenhouse. Allspice berries are picked while still green and unripe, then dried in the sun, turning purple and then brown in the process. They resemble peppercorns in appearance but are bigger and lighter in colour, with a rough surface consisting of volatile oil glands, and two hard seeds inside.

19

BUYING AND STORING

It is best to buy whole berries and grind them as needed to conserve their flavour. If stored in an airtight container kept out of direct sunlight, allspice berries should keep for several years.

FOOD PROFILE

Allspice is an integral part of Caribbean cuisine, adding a warm, rich flavour to many traditional dishes, particularly soups, stews and curries. Since its arrival in Europe, allspice has also become an important part of European, Mediterranean, Middle Eastern, Indian and American cuisines, and is a popular ingredient in baking, pickling and preserving; for sausages, herring, mincemeat, cakes and cookies; in spice mixtures; and in liqueurs and wines. It is also commonly used in the food industry in sauces and preserves.

NUTRITIONAL PROFILE

Allspice has a pungent, peppery flavour and contains antioxidant phenols, including eugenol, in its volatile oil. Eugenol, which is also found in cloves, is both antioxidant and antimicrobial, and is an effective antiseptic and local anaesthetic.

HEALTH PROFILE

With its warming, relaxing and opening quality, allspice can be used to relieve indigestion, diarrhoea and wind, and to treat infections. It is also used in the manufacture of deodorants and some perfumes.

Amchoor *Mangifera indica*

Mango powder, known variously as amchoor, amchor, aamchur and amchur, is a popular northeast Indian spice made from dried, green, extremely tart, unripe mangoes. The green mangoes, grown on evergreen tropical trees that can live for well over 100 years, are sliced and dried in the sun before being ground down to a fine powder. Amchoor has a sweet and sour quality and, just like a ripe mango, is packed full of health-enhancing phytochemicals.

BUYING AND STORING

Amchoor is available in most Asian stores and markets as a grey or golden powder, depending on how much turmeric has been added. Stored in an airtight container in a cool, dry place, out of direct sunlight, amchoor will keep for up to a year.

FOOD PROFILE

Amchoor has a tangy, sour, slightly fruity flavour, similar to tamarind, and is used as a thickening, tenderizing spice, especially in northern Indian cuisine. It is a traditional ingredient in masalas and jalfrezis, soups, curries, chutneys and condiments, as well as in spiced drinks. It also works well in marinades for grills and barbecues, and tastes excellent sprinkled on roast potatoes.

NUTRITIONAL PROFILE

Unripe mango is rich in vitamins A and C, giving amchoor strong antioxidant qualities. It also contains several other antioxidants (including magniferin, phenols, lupeol, quercetin, kaempferol and gallic acid) as well as tannins and essential nutrients such as pyridoxine (B6), folate, potassium, copper and amino and omega acids.

HEALTH PROFILE

Lupeol has been shown to protect cells against inflammation, pollution and the development of cancers (especially of the skin and prostate gland) by mopping up free radicals and blocking DNA mutation. A possible protective effect on thyroid function and cardiovascular health has also been reported.

NOTE:

* Amchoor can be used to replace vinegar, lime, tamarind or lemon juice in many recipes.

Aniseed 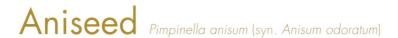 *Pimpinella anisum* (syn. *Anisum odoratum*)

Also known as anise and sweet cumin, aniseed is a herbaceous annual plant native to the eastern Mediterranean and southwest Asia. It is a member of the parsley family (*Apiaceae*) that consists of over 3,000 different species, including carrot and parsley. Aniseed is easily identified by its sweet, aromatic, liquorice-like flavour, which is strongest in the seeds, but also present in the leaves. The plant has a long history of culinary and medicinal use, and is cultivated in many parts of the world because it is easy to grow and resows itself every year once established. Aniseed prefers light, well-drained soil and warm, sheltered locations.

BUYING AND STORING

Aniseeds are sold whole, cracked or powdered, and are sometimes confused with fennel seeds (which are larger, paler and less aromatic). As with most spices, it is best to buy whole seeds and use them whole, or crushed in a mortar only as needed, because they release their flavour and aroma as soon as they are ground. Stored in an airtight container, out of direct sunlight, whole aniseeds retain their flavour for several years.

FOOD PROFILE

Aniseed has a long history of culinary use in both savoury and sweet dishes and drinks. It is used commercially to flavour cakes, cookies and confectionery, and also in anise-flavoured aperitifs, the most famous of which is Pernod. Aniseed leaves have a milder flavour and can be added fresh to salads, or scattered on cooked dishes. The flavour of the seeds is enhanced by toasting.

NUTRITIONAL PROFILE

The main components of aniseed are volatile oils, particularly anethole.

HEALTH PROFILE

Anethole is a phytoestrogen that shares structural similarities with adrenaline and dopamine, which explains the traditional use of aniseed in the treatment of asthma, to promote weight loss and to increase milk flow in nursing mothers. It has also been used to treat menstrual cramps, constipation, colic, flatulence and indigestion, as a cure for sleeplessness and bad breath, and externally to get rid of lice and scabies infestations. Anise oil is also used in soaps, perfumes, confectionery and cough remedies.

Asafoetida *Ferula asafoetida*

Native to southwest Asia and the mountains of Iran and Afghanistan, asafoetida is now cultivated mainly in India. Like aniseed, it is in the parsely family (*Apiaceae*) and a perennial herb that grows up to 2m/6ft high.

The whole plant gives off a pungent, almost fetid smell, which can be distinctly unpleasant and quite overpowering (hence the common name 'devil's dung'). The odour comes from a resin found in the sap, which is extracted from the root, then dried and made into a powder. The sulphurous smell of asafoetida powder is reminiscent of a mixture of onion and garlic, and sometimes it replaces these ingredients in Indian cooking. Used sparingly, the powder has a mild sweet flavour when cooked, and it can enhance the taste of a variety dishes (which could be the reason for its other common name, 'food of the gods').

BUYING AND STORING

The dried resin is sold in solid lumps and pastes, but the easiest way to buy and store it is as a yellow powder, which is usually sold in sealed tubs. Asafoetida powder is often mixed with flour and turmeric to give more bulk, and one small, well-sealed, airtight tub will keep its flavour and odour for months, or even years.

FOOD PROFILE

To use asafoetida as a natural flavour enhancer, heat a pinch of powder in a little oil along with any other spices before adding other ingredients. It works well added to curries and stews, pickles, fritters, grills and marinades, and is an essential flavouring in Worcestershire sauce.

NUTRITIONAL PROFILE

Asafoetida contains resins, gums and a volatile oil rich in polyphenols.

HEALTH PROFILE

Once famous for its use in fighting the Spanish flu pandemic of 1918, asafoetida is a powerful antiviral, antioxidant and antimicrobial. It has been used to treat respiratory infections, bronchitis, whooping cough and asthma, and its ability to relax smooth muscle makes it useful in the relief of intestinal cramping and flatulence.

NOTE:
- Try growing your own asafoetida: the leaves and young shoots can be cooked and served as a tender vegetable, like spinach.

Bay Leaf *Laurus nobilis*

The slow-growing bay tree thrives in hedges, sunny borders and by south-facing walls, and its leaves (also known as sweet bay, bay laurel or victor's laurel) have a warm, pungent and slightly bitter taste. They are most often used dried to add their aromatic flavour to soups, stews, bakes and casseroles, and are an essential ingredient of the court bouillon and bouquet garni of European and Mediterranean cooking.

Fresh bay leaves have a sharp, bitter taste, which matures on drying to a far more aromatic flavour. Like most spices, bay leaves are best added at the beginning of the cooking process (whereas herbs are usually added toward the end) so their complex flavour has time to infuse and blend with all the ingredients.

BUYING AND STORING

Slow-dried bay leaves are more aromatic than fresh (which can have an unpleasantly sharp and bitter flavour), and keep best if stored in an airtight container out of direct sunlight. Try to buy dusky, dark green leaves, avoiding small, pale or yellowed ones, and discard them after a year as their flavour diminishes with age.

FOOD PROFILE

Use dried whole bay leaves sparingly as their flavour can be quite overpowering; often one is enough for a dish. Always remember to remove any bay leaves from dishes before serving as they remain hard even after cooking and are unpleasant to chew and swallow. Crushed bay leaves do impart more flavour but they are best used in a muslin/cheesecloth bag for easy removal after cooking. An excellent addition to soups, stews, stir-fries and sauces, bay leaves are also a common ingredient in a wide range of marinades and pickles, and can add a lightly spicy, aromatic flavour to sweet custards and creamy desserts.

NUTRITIONAL PROFILE

Bay leaves contain volatile oils, myrcene, cineole and eugenol, as well as sesquiterpenes, parthenolide and oleic and linoleic acid. Freshly dried older leaves and young stems have the highest oil content.

HEALTH PROFILE

The ancient Greeks held bay leaves in high esteem for their medicinal value, and to this day they are used by herbalists for their antibacterial, antifungal, antiviral and strong antioxidant properties. They have been shown to boost insulin sensitivity and to help lower blood cholesterol. Recent studies suggest that bay leaves may also inhibit the growth of cancer cells.

Bay leaves can also be used as a natural insecticide, a worming remedy and as a mosquito repellent.

NOTES:
- Try an invigorating bath-time treat by adding a muslin/cheesecloth bag full of crushed bay leaves to your bath as you run the hot water.
- Bay leaves can be kept in storage jars to repel food moths.

Black Cumin *Bunium persicum*

Black cumin is often confused with *kalonji* (nigella seed/*Nigella sativa*), as described on page 69. It is also known as black seed, black cumin, Kashmiri cumin, *gov-zira* or *kala zeera*, and it is synonymous with (or very closely related to) *Bunium bulbocastanum*, which is also known as great pignut or earth chestnut.

Black cumin seeds are ridged and similar to caraway in shape, although they are longer and narrower. The plant, another member of the parsley family (*Apiaceae*), is a perennial with an edible, tuber-like tap root, and grows up to 60cm/2ft tall with green feathery leaves and white flower umbels. It is native to the mountains of Central Asia, where it can be found on dry, exposed grassy slopes, but it is now naturalized in southeastern Europe, Central and South Asia and northern India, where it is grown commercially, especially in Kashmir.

BUYING AND STORING

As the taste of black cumin depends on the volatile oils contained in the seeds, it is advisable to buy whole seeds and grind them as needed to avoid any loss of flavour. Store the seeds in an airtight container out of direct sunlight and use within a year.

FOOD PROFILE

Black cumin is popular in northern Indian, Arabian and Caucasian cuisine, but there has long been confusion between black cumin and nigella seeds, which, although quite different in appearance, are both called black cumin in some local languages. Much valued in Moghul cooking (which is known for its heavy use of aromatic spices, dried fruit and rich sauces), black cumin adds a pleasant, slightly sweet, nutty flavour to dishes and drinks. It is one of the key ingredients in the traditional Bengali spice mixture Panch Phoron (see page 115).

NUTRITIONAL PROFILE

Rich in volatile oils including p-mentha, terpinene and cuminaldehyde, studies show that black cumin has a strong antihistaminic and bronchodilatory effect.

HEALTH PROFILE

Traditionally, the seeds have been used for relieving diarrhoea and indigestion, and black cumin tisane has been shown to lower blood sugar, making it helpful in the management of type-2 diabetes and obesity. The essential oil has a history of use in Ayurvedic medicine for digestive problems, infections and, externally, for injuries, bruises and boils.

Caraway Seeds *Carum carvi*

Caraway seeds are the small, brown, crescent-shaped seeds of a 50cm/20in tall, hardy biennial plant that has white flower umbels and finely feathered leaves. Also known as Persian cumin, caraway is native to western Asia and North Africa, and was later introduced to northern and central Europe and America. The plant thrives in light, well-drained soils and sunny positions. It is best sown in situ as it has a large tap root, which can make it difficult to move once established. It produces seeds in the second year of growth. Like the other aromatic members of the parsely family (*Apiaceae*), notably dill, fennel and aniseed, caraway has been been valued as a spice and a medicine for centuries. The leaves and seeds have a pleasant aromatic scent and flavour, and the seeds have a pungent, sharp, anise-like taste.

BUYING AND STORING

The seeds are harvested as soon as they begin to turn dark and should be stored in an airtight container out of direct sunlight. As with most other spices, to achieve the fullest flavour, it is best to buy whole seeds and grind them only as required.

FOOD PROFILE

The whole caraway plant is edible, but only the seeds are used as a spice. They have a sharp, almost liquorice taste and are popular additions to cheeses, sauerkraut and sausages. They are also commonly used to add interesting flavour to baked fruits, cakes, rolls and Scandinavian breads. The young leaves taste good in soups and salads, and the root can be cooked and eaten like parsnip. The popular German liqueur Kümmel is flavoured with caraway.

NUTRITIONAL PROFILE

Caraway contains a number of volatile oils, including carvone, limonene and a type of camphor. It also contains resin, coumarin, fatty oil and tannin.

HEALTH PROFILE

Caraway has a reputation in traditional medicine for easing indigestion and wind, and a weak tisane made from the seeds (perhaps sweetened with a little honey) can be an excellent remedy for childhood colic. Caraway can be combined with fennel to promote milk flow in nursing mothers (with the added advantage of calming the baby's digestion), and can also act as a mild painkiller. New research indicates a role for caraway in the management of auto-immune thyroid problems such as Hashimoto's disease. The essential oil is used in cosmetics, soaps, creams, perfumes and lotions.

Cardamom *Elettaria cardamomum*

Sometimes known as the 'queen of spice', true cardamom is one of the world's most valued and expensive spices, only surpassed in price by vanilla and saffron. The cardamom plant is native to the mountain rainforests of southern India and Sri Lanka, although today it is widely cultivated on large-scale plantations from India to Malaysia, and in Sri Lanka, Vietnam, Tanzania and Guatemala.

The valued green seedpods come from certain varieties of the *Elettaria* genera of the ginger family (*Zingiberaceae*) but buying true cardamom can be confusing because other related cardamoms are available from the *Amomum* and *Aframomum* species, which also belong to the ginger family. Varieties of *Amomum* are native to Nepal and the eastern Himalayas and include the inferior cardamom substitutes known as black cardamom, Bengal cardamom, Nepal cardamom, greater cardamom, winged cardamom and brown cardamom. Their seedpods look similar to those of green cardamom, but are larger, darker and coarser. These seeds have a strong, camphor-like, smoky cardamom taste, partly because traditionally they are dried over open fires. The stronger-flavoured varieties are widely used in Chinese, Vietnamese and African cooking, and are also sold as cheap substitutes for the more highly valued and aromatic green cardamoms.

BUYING AND STORING

Cardamom is available as whole pods, loose seeds and in powder form. The seeds quickly lose the intensity of their flavour once the pods are opened, so it is always best to buy whole pods and extract the seeds as required. Each pod contains 10–20 tiny, highly aromatic, dark brown or black seeds, which smell sharp and lemony.

FOOD PROFILE

Cardamom is widely used in Indian dishes, sweet as well as savoury, and is popular in Scandinavia for flavouring breads and cakes, notably Christmas cakes. In Asian and Middle Eastern cookery, cardamom is often used in desserts and added to coffee and tea to enhance their fragrance. All the flavouring is in the tiny black seeds and only a small quantity is required to impart their unique, fresh lemony taste.

NUTRITIONAL PROFILE

Cardamom seeds contain up to 8% volatile oil including terpineol, myrcene, limonene, menthone, eucalyptol (1,8-cineol) and borneol.

HEALTH PROFILE

In traditional Chinese and Indian medicine, cardamom has long been valued as a treatment for a range of digestive and respiratory disorders as well as malaria. It is known to be strongly antiseptic and can be chewed like gum to treat mouth and gum infections and freshen the breath. Cardamom is thought to calm intestinal peristalsis, inhibit stomach ulcers and reduce inflammation and cancer cell proliferation in the large intestines, which supports its traditional use as a warming, soothing digestive remedy to relieve colic. Some people find that cardamom can also ease acid reflux.

NOTE:
• The seeds of seven whole cardamom pods are equivalent to 1 teaspoon of ground cardamom.

Cassia *Cinnamomum cassia*

Also referred to as Chinese cinnamon, Canton cassia and bastard cinnamon, cassia is the bark of a tall evergreen tree native to the hills along the border between southern China and Myanmar. It is an ancient spice, valued in China as a medicine and flavouring for 5,000 years or more. Its use is also recorded in the Bible and other classical texts. The cassia tree belongs to the laurel family (*Lauraceae*), and has a greyish outer bark that covers the inner, deep rust-red cassia bark. This curls slightly as it dries, and though it is quite similar to cinnamon, cassia is harder, coarser and more difficult to crush. It is generally considered inferior as a spice to its relative, true cinnamon (see pages 35–37), and is less expensive, although it has a sweeter, stronger flavour.

BUYING AND STORING

In North America, cassia is widely sold as cinnamon, while in other parts of the world it can only be labelled as cassia. In Europe, cassia is available in Asian food stores.

FOOD PROFILE

Cassia tastes very similar to cinnamon, but its flavour is less delicate and slightly astringent. It has a warm, intense quality and is commonly used whole as an aroma enhancer in savoury dishes, especially with braised meats; grains such as rice, couscous and barley; split peas and lentils. Cassia is also commonly used for pickling and in spice mixtures, desserts, curries and chocolate. It is an essential spice in Chinese cuisine and a constituent of Chinese five-spice powder (see page 117).

NUTRITIONAL PROFILE

Cassia contains volatile oil, cinnamaldehyde, coumarin, diterpenes, catechins, proanthocyanidins and tannins.

HEALTH PROFILE

Like cinnamon, cassia can be used to relieve colic, wind and diarrhoea, and in traditional Chinese medicine it is thought of as a pure yang herb that disperses cold, supports yang and alleviates pain. It has a relatively high coumarin content, which gives it anticoagulant properties. It also contains cinnamaldehyde, which is a natural antibacterial and antifungal remedy, and may have a blood-sugar-lowering effect.

WARNING:

- Cassia should never be eaten in large amounts and should always be used with caution during pregnancy.
- As cassia may affect the action of anti-diabetic medication, consult your physician on including cassia in your diet if you are diabetic.

Celery Seed *Apium graveolens*

Native to the eastern Mediterranean region, the tiny seeds of wild celery were valued and praised as a food and medicine in ancient Egyptian and Greek cultures. The wild celery plant belongs to the parsley family (*Apiaceae*), and is a biennial, growing to 1m/3ft tall with feathery leaves that resemble flat parsley but with a distinctive celery smell. The flowers sit in dense, creamy-white umbels and the seeds are tiny, egg-shaped, light brown and ridged, with a pungent celery aroma reminiscent of new-mown hay. Wild celery can be found in damp habitats by rivers, and in marshes and ditches, especially near the sea.

BUYING AND STORING

Whole seeds keep better than ground, and can be used as they are or crushed to a coarse powder only when required. Toasting the seeds first helps to bring out their unique, sweet flavour.

FOOD PROFILE

Celery seeds go well with tomatoes, carrots and salads, and are excellent in soups, stews and casseroles. They also add an interesting flavour to breads and cookies, but be sparing; their strong taste can easily become overpowering.

NUTRITIONAL PROFILE

Celery seeds contain apiol and coumarins, and are a good source of iron, phosphorus, potassium and sodium.

HEALTH PROFILE

Long-used in traditional medicine as a blood purifier, celery seed is thought to make the blood more alkaline. It is also thought to help the body eliminate uric acid, and is considered an anti-rheumatic, diuretic and urinary antiseptic remedy effective in the management of gout, cystitis and kidney stones. Celery seeds have a reputation for increasing milk flow in nursing mothers and for promoting sleep.

NOTES:
- Celery salt, made by grinding equal amounts of celery seed and salt together, is a useful condiment to help reduce sodium intake.
- A Virgin Mary cocktail, made from tomato juice, lemon juice, celery salt, pepper, Tabasco, and Worcestershire sauce (optional), is a refreshing drink that may lessen the effect of a hangover.

WARNING:
- Celery seed can cause allergic reactions in people with a history of hypersensitivity.

CHILLI PEPPERS *Capsicum annuum,*
Capsicum baccatum, Capsicum frutescens, Capsicum pubescens
and species

Native to Central and South America, chillies were introduced to South Asia
by Portuguese traders in the 16th century and were soon adopted as essential
ingredients. India is now the largest producer, consumer and exporter of chillies,
followed by Mexico, China, Indonesia and Thailand.

The chilli pepper comes from a genus of perennial plants belonging to the
nightshade family (*Solanaceae*). After flowering, the capsicum plants bear green,
brown, yellow, orange or red peppery fruits, depending on the maturity of flavour
and pungency desired. These all contain capsaicin, which gives them a characteristic
hot, sweet, fruity flavour that becomes more complex when the fruits are dried.

The hotness of chillies is measured in 'Scoville Units' (after Wilbur Scoville,
a pharmacist who developed the test in 1912). Scores range from zero (for
the sweet bell pepper) to over a million (for the hottest chilli record-breakers),
depending on the amount of capsaicin they contain.

Here is a selection of the most popular chillies from more than 400 types grown
around the world:

Aji Amarillo – very hot, yellowish-orange Peruvian chilli.

Aji Cereza – extremely hot wild Peruvian chilli, resembling a cherry.

Aji Limo – even hotter South American chilli, with a distinct berry-like taste, deep red colour
and lantern shape.

Aji Mirasol – very hot, yellowish-red, 10cm/4in-long Peruvian chilli.

Aji Panca – relatively mild Peruvian chilli with a berry-like taste.

Aji Pinguita – extremely hot, small, pointed, red Peruvian chilli.

Aleppo/Halaby Pepper – robust, burnt-red chilli from the Syrian city of Aleppo. Gentle
but deeply aromatic and sweet, it has an almost smoky heat, high oil content and a slow release
of hotness.

Anaheim – relatively mild green or red, 15cm/6in-long Californian chilli. Also known as
Colorado chilli.

Ancho – a flat, large, heart-shaped, sweet, fruity, hot Mexican chilli.

Arbol – very hot, narrow, 5–7cm/2–2¾in-long chilli, bright green to bright red. Also known as bird's beak chilli, Thai chilli or cayenne, it is available fresh, dried and powdered, and keeps its colour when dried.

Cascabel – plum-shaped, dark red, medium-hot chilli that has a rich nutty flavour. Also known as chilli bola.

Cayenne – from the French Guianan region of Cayenne, an extremely hot, long, thin, pointed, red/brown chilli with a distinctive flavour. Usually dried and ground to a fine powder, made from seeds and pods.

Charleston Hot – cayenne type, but much hotter, 10–12cm/4–4½in long, ripening from green to yellow and orange.

Cherry – round and red, mild to moderately hot, chilli.

Dundicut – spherical or teardrop-shaped, ruby-red, fruity and very hot chilli from Pakistan.

Habanero – South American; one of the world's hottest and most fiery chillies. It matures from green to yellow, red and brown.

Jalapeño – one of the best-known hot chilli peppers; 5cm/2in long, tapered, green or red, it is often available canned or pickled. When it has been dried and smoked, it is called a chipotle.

Macho – extremely hot, intensely fiery and sharp, small, light green to red Mexican chilli.

Mirasol – hot, 7cm/2¾in, bright red, pointed Mexican chilli, which has a strawberry-like taste.

Mulato – mild, 10–15cm/4–6in, dark-chocolate-coloured, smoky liquorice-flavoured Mexican chilli.

Paprika – mild to hot with warm, sweet flavour (see pages 73–74).

Pasilla – relatively mild, dark green to purple Mexican chilli with a smoky flavour.

Pequin – the smallest, but one of the hottest, round or conical-shaped chillies. Adds fire and flavour to salsas, sauces and pickles.

Peter Pepper – rare, hot, red or green, phallus-shaped Texan chilli.

Pepperoncini – mild red chilli, also known as Tuscan Pepper.

Poblano – mild to hot, very dark green, with tapering bell shape. This is the most popular Mexican chilli.

Red Savina Habanero – held the record as the hottest chilli for many years; red, Chinese-lantern-shaped with an intense, burning heat.

Rocoto – very hot, egg-shaped, orange-red Mexican chilli that has big black seeds. Usually used fresh to make salsas.

Scotch Bonnet – extremely hot Caribbean chilli, also known as Jamaican Hot or Martinique

Pepper. Closely related to the Habanero, similar in shape, but smaller. Used for sauces, marinades and salsas.

Serrano – very hot, small, green or red torpedo-shaped chilli from the mountains of Mexico. Used in salsas and sauces.

Tabasco – very hot, bright red, small chilli that grows upward on the plant. Used to make Tabasco sauce.

Tepin – also known as Chiltepin. A tiny, very hot, bright red, wild South American berry, thought to be the ancestor of all chillies.

Tien Tsin – small, very hot, bright red Chinese chilli. Used whole or added to chilli oil in Asian cuisine.

Tōgarashi – small, very hot, red Japanese chilli. The name means 'Chinese mustard'. Used fresh or dried.

Wax – a group of shiny chillies of varying heat, size, shape and colour.

BUYING AND STORING

Fresh chillies should be smooth, firm and glossy, and will keep for 2–3 weeks in the refrigerator or 6 months in the freezer. Store dried and ground chillies in an airtight jar out of direct sunlight.

FOOD PROFILE

Hot chillies must be handled with great care. Consider wearing surgical gloves, or wash your hands immediately after touching them. Above all, avoid contact with your eyes and other sensitive parts of the body. Use chillies, fresh or dried, in curries, sauces, casseroles, pickles, chutneys, pastes and dips to add heat and sweetness. Removing the seeds will reduce some of their hotness. Be careful not to use more than you need: it is hard to undo the effect of chilli in a dish, although coconut milk, peanut butter, cream, yogurt or sugar can tone down the heat a little.

NUTRITIONAL PROFILE

Chillies are very high in vitamins A and C, E, K and B6, and contain capsaicin (in varying amounts), carotenoids and steroidal saponins.

HEALTH PROFILE

Chilli stimulates the heart and circulation, increasing blood flow to the tissues, producing a natural warmth and increased metabolism. It is also antioxidant with anti-inflammatory properties, and can be used as a natural antiseptic, digestive stimulant and food preservative. Chilli is an effective external remedy for minor muscle and joint pain, decreasing the volume of pain signals sent to the brain. Capsaicin may help to lower blood cholesterol and is also a natural anticoagulant, so hot chillies should be avoided when taking such medication. Recent research indicates that chilli may provoke endorphin release in the brain, creating a sense of pleasure and wellbeing.

NOTES:
- Try peeling and slicing an orange, sprinkling the slices with cayenne pepper and sugar, then grilling/broiling them.
- Using whole chillies, instead of sliced or ground, will add flavour to a dish without too much heat. Remember to remove before serving.
- To remove their skins, grill/broil fresh chillies until black and charred, then cool in a paper bag. The skins should peel off easily.
- To cool a burning mouth caused by too much chilli, eat something soft and sweet, starchy or creamy: try bread, rice, sugar, peanut butter, yogurt or milk.

CINNAMON *Cinnamomum verum*

True cinnamon quills are made from the inner bark of a small, bushy evergreen tree, native to the forests of southern India and Sri Lanka. In Europe, the name refers only to *Cinnamomum verum*, which produces bark that is much thinner than cassia, with pale tan quills rolled inside each other, but around 250 species of the *Cinnamomum* genus of the laurel family (*Lauraceae*) produce cinnamon-like quills, notably cassia (see pages 29–30); in America, several other *cinnamomum* species are classed as cinnamon.

Cinnamon is one of the oldest-known aromatic spices, the first record of use being in China around 2800 BC. Many cultures have enjoyed the power and beauty of cinnamon, from the Egyptians to the Phoenicians and the Hebrews, who all mention it in their writings. It reached Europe in the 1st century AD but was very hard to come by and, for a time, became more expensive than gold. When the Dutch took Sri Lanka from the Portuguese in the 17th century, their monopoly of the cinnamon trade made the spice more widely available. The old botanical name,

C. zeylanicum, reflects cinnamon's origins in Sri Lanka, which was known as Ceylon. Almost 90% of this remarkable and delicate spice is still produced there, with the rest coming from the islands of Madagascar, Mauritius, the Seychelles and the West Indies.

BUYING AND STORING

The best cinnamon quills are smooth, light brown and paper-thin. Choose whole sticks because cinnamon soon loses some of its sweet, warming aroma once ground. Store in an airtight jar away from direct sunlight.

FOOD PROFILE

With its sweet, warm, pungent, aromatic taste and an unmistakable, sweetly exotic, woody aroma, cinnamon is used in countless cuisines, and the addition of whole quills imparts a rich flavour to stir-fries, stews and soups; rice and lentil dishes; desserts and drinks. Ground cinnamon adds a sweet, comforting flavour to fruit salads and smoothies, and is used extensively in breads, chocolate, cakes and spice mixtures. Mixing ground cinnamon with a little sugar and sprinkling it over rice puddings, pancakes and milky desserts is a popular tradition in many parts of the world.

NUTRITIONAL PROFILE

Cinnamon contains essential oil, tannins, coumarin, calcium, iron and vitamin K.

HEALTH PROFILE

A warming spice with sedative, antispasmodic, antibacterial and antifungal properties, cinnamon is useful in the treatment of digestive problems and can also help to stimulate the appetite. As well as relieving nausea, vomiting, diarrhoea and stomach cramps, it is used traditionally as a remedy for colds, flu, arthritis and high blood pressure. Contemporary evidence confirms that cinnamon helps to lower blood pressure and increases peripheral blood flow.

Cinnamon's antibacterial and antifungal properties are also supported by research. Clinical trials have shown cinnamon to be effective against oral thrush; new research shows that, when taken regularly over a period of time, cinnamon can help to improve insulin sensitivity and reduce high blood sugar and high cholesterol. With type-2 diabetes becoming an increasing problem worldwide, the fact that cinnamon has been shown to reduce glucose absorption by inhibiting pancreatic secretions, and that it is capable of stimulating glucose uptake into cells by promoting insulin release and activity, could be of great significance.

Cinnamon also has immune-boosting antioxidant and anti-inflammatory properties, which may be effective in cancer prevention. It is also used in the manufacture of cosmetics, mouthwashes and other pharmaceutical products.

NOTES:
- Vary the flavour of a hot drink by stirring it with a cinnamon quill.
- Cinnamon sugar is easy to make at home: put 3 tablespoons of sugar and 1 teaspoon of ground cinnamon into a jar, seal and shake well.

WARNING:
- Use with caution during pregnancy and in cases of stomach ulcers.
- Large doses may cause allergic skin reactions.

CLOVES *Syzygium aromaticum*

Native to the Banda Islands in the Moluccas, Indonesia, cloves are the unopened, dried flower buds of the clove tree. The name comes from *clavus*, the Latin word for nail, and refers to the shape of the unopened flower bud. The clove tree is an evergreen that grows 12m/39ft tall and belongs to the myrtle family (*Myrtaceae*). After about eight years, the tree starts to bear fruit. The cloves are picked when green and dried in the sun until they turn brown-black and fill the warm air with the smell of Christmas cake and carnations.

Cloves were once extremely highly valued in the food and pharmaceutical industries for both their flavour and their unique medicinal qualities. First mentioned in ancient Chinese texts (visitors to the Chinese court chewed cloves to avoid offending the Emperor with their bad breath), cloves are thought to have been imported into China from the Spice Islands more than 2,000 years ago. Many years later, the spice became popular in Europe and, together with nutmeg, brought huge rewards to successful spice merchants in the East Indian and Spice Island trade. Indeed, for many years, cloves were worth their own weight in gold.

Cloves were also responsible for the presence on the Spice Islands of the

Portuguese, who had a clove-trade monopoly for 60 years. This ended in 1605 when the Dutch took possession of the islands and destroyed all the clove trees, except those on one solitary, remote and well-guarded island called Ambon, thus taking total control of all the clove trade (and the price) for 200 years. During this time, any person caught carrying or growing cloves or seedlings without permission could be put to death. It was the French missionary and horticulturalist, Pierre Poivre (better known in English as Peter Piper) who, according to legend, managed to steal and smuggle fresh clove buds from the secret island and transplant them on Mauritius.

Clove-mania continued and soon this remarkable spice was established and being grown successfully in other parts of the world. Today, clove trees are found throughout the tropics, from sea-level up to 600m/1,968ft, notably in Brazil, French Guiana, the Caribbean, India, Indonesia, the Philippines, Sumatra, Madagascar, Tanzania and Zanzibar. Interestingly, nothing from the tree is wasted: the whole buds are used for spice; the stems and broken buds for oil; and the leaves for fuel.

BUYING AND STORING

Look for whole buds with a dark, reddish-brown colour, no sign of white flakes or insect bore holes. Oil should seep out when the bud is pressed with a fingernail. Use whole cloves, or grind only as required.

FOOD PROFILE

Cloves are popular throughout the Middle East, Africa and Asia in curries, casseroles and marinades, as well as in coffees, teas, pilau rice and many different spice blends. Cloves are also popular in the West to flavour desserts and pies, and to add aroma to roasts, sauces, stocks, stews and drinks. They have a strong flavour, however, and should always be used sparingly.

NUTRITIONAL PROFILE

Cloves contain at least 15% volatile oil, particularly eugenol, which is an effective antiseptic and local anaesthetic. Cloves also contain methyl salycilate, salicylic acid, camphor resin, flavonols and sterols.

HEALTH PROFILE

Cloves have long been used in dentistry for local anaesthesia. They also have a history of use as a dental antiseptic with antibacterial and antifungal properties, and as a mouthwash to relieve gum disease and toothache. They are also used in traditional herbal medicine to calm digestive problems, relieve cramps and help in the treatment of 'cold' conditions. Research has found that eugenol does bring heat and stimulates digestive secretions, thus aiding digestion and relieving cramps and wind.

Modern research suggests that clove oil can be taken as an alternative to aspirin in preventing the formation of blood clots, and that cloves can help to increase insulin activity and lower the body's blood sugar levels. Cloves are known to have strong antioxidant properties, helping to boost the immune system. They have proved effective in treatments against the infection *Helicobacter pylori* (linked to the formation of stomach ulcers and, possibly, gastric cancer), as well as *E. coli*, and as an antiviral remedy they may inhibit the growth of herpes simplex, hepatitis C, HIV and some of the viruses that can cause leukaemia.

Clove oil is usually diluted in a carrier oil, such as almond, and can be a good remedy for dry skin. It is a natural insect repellent and is found in a number of bio-pesticides.

NOTES:

- Cloves go well with prunes, plums, apple, rice and dal.
- Increase the rich intensity of a sauce, soup or stew by adding a whole peeled onion studded with cloves to the mixture.
- A thin-skinned orange stuck with cloves and rolled in orris root makes an effective room freshener.

WARNING:

- Concentrated clove oil can be toxic in large doses. Always use sparingly

Cocoa *Theobroma cacao*

Native to the tropical forests of southeastern Mexico and the foothills of the Andes, cocoa was sacred to the ancient Mayan and Aztec civilizations, and *Theobroma*, the Latin name for the cocoa bean, translates as 'food of the gods'.

The cocoa bean is the seed of an evergreen tropical tree belonging to the mallow family (*Malvaceae*). The cocoa, or cacao, tree grows up to 10m/32ft tall and produces long, entire leaves and clusters of small creamy-yellow flowers with pink calyxes borne directly on the trunk and branches. The flowers develop into large green, red or puple egg-shaped fruit pods, that turn yellow to orange as they ripen. Each pod weighs about 500g/1lb 2oz and contains 30–50 large soft white seeds, known as beans. After harvesting, the beans are fermented and dried for export and processing.

The cocoa tree is now widely grown throughout southeastern Mexico and the Amazon region. It is also grown in countries within the world's tropical regions, including the West Indies, Asia and West Africa, which now produces most of the world's cocoa crop. The global production of cocoa has more than doubled in the past 30 years.

BUYING AND STORING

Over 4 million tonnes of cocoa beans are produced and consumed in the world each year and chocolate, in its many and various forms, is now available almost everywhere.

Whole cocoa beans (if ever you have them) can be stored for several years. Cocoa powder, stored in a dry and relatively cool place, does not go off, but the flavour decreases over time so it is best used within a couple of years.

FOOD PROFILE

Cocoa powder is made from ground cocoa beans from which the cocoa butter has been removed. It is not the same as chocolate powder, which also contains sugar and dried milk. To make 100g/3½oz of chocolate requires 30–60 roasted cocoa beans, cocoa butter, sugar and, sometimes, an emulsifier (lecithin). Cocoa butter is also used in the manufacture of confectionery and in cosmetics.

NUTRITIONAL PROFILE

Cocoa contains theobromine (a stimulant similar to caffeine), caffeine, tyramine, anandamide, flavonoids, procyanidins and a high percentage of fixed oil (cocoa butter), as well as vitamins B2, B3 and tryptophan, calcium, iron, magnesium, zinc, copper and selenium. Roasting has a degrading effect on the flavonoid content of cocoa.

HEALTH PROFILE

Cocoa is antioxidant, nourishing and mildly diuretic. It stimulates endorphine release, which creates a sense of inner comfort and wellbeing, and also aids serotonin production, which can have a beneficial effect on mood. Overall, cocoa is thought to have a protective effect on the heart and circulation, and it contains monounsaturated fat, which may help to lower blood cholesterol levels.

Chocolate is less healthy than cocoa because it also contains fat and sugar and is more calorie-dense. Although dark/bittersweet chocolate, with its high cocoa content, is healthier than milk chocolate, it still contains sugar and should be enjoyed in moderation.

NOTE:

- It has been estimated that there are as many as 200,000 enslaved children working on cocoa farms in Africa. Buying organic or Fairtrade chocolate is one way to avoid supporting such practice.

Coriander *Coriandrum sativum*

Native to the Middle East, coriander was cultivated by the Babylonians as long ago as 800 BC. By 200 BC it had spread as far as China. Since then it has been naturalized all over Europe, North Africa, Asia and North and South America and is cultivated worldwide. Its culinary and medicinal attributes have been documented for over 3,000 years and such is its significance that it was one of the earliest spice plants to be introduced by settlers to North America.

Also known as *cilantro*, *dhania*, Arabian parsley and Chinese parsley, coriander is an annual herbaceous plant that grows up to 50cm/20in tall. It belongs to the parsley family (*Apiaceae*) and has broadly lobed aromatic leaves and forms white or pastel pink flowers arranged in asymmetrical umbels.

Coriander seeds are the dried ripe fruits that look like pale golden peppercorns. All parts of the coriander plant can be used as food and medicine, and the fresh plant has a distinctive, pungent aroma, which is loved by some and hated by others. The ripe, dry seeds have a milder, sweeter almost woody scent and a warming, soft flavour.

BUYING AND STORING

Buy whole coriander seeds and store them in an airtight container out of direct sunlight. Grind them only as required, rather than buying them as a ready-ground powder, and toast them first to bring out their full flavour. The leaves of the coriander plant are best used fresh, although it is possible to buy them freeze-dried.

FOOD PROFILE

The fresh leaves and stems of coriander (cilantro) impart their distinctive flavour to the foods of South Asia, South America and the Middle East. The seeds are one of the world's most popular spices and are commonly used to flavour curries, stews, stir-fries, sausages, breads, confectionery and condiments, and for pickling and brewing.

NUTRITIONAL PROFILE

Coriander seeds contain essential oils together with camphor, linalol, geraniol, terpenes, flavonoids, coumarins, phenolic acids, sterols and omega oils.

HEALTH PROFILE

Coriander has been taken to treat indigestion, wind, colic and cramps, and to stimulate the appetite since ancient times. More recently it has been recommended in the management of type-2 diabetes and as a diuretic. It is thought to reduce the uptake of heavy metals from the diet, and may even help to remove them from the body. It is also thought to reduce the effect of ulcerogenic *Helicobacter pylori* infection, and has been shown to be effective against both gram-positive and gram-negative bacteria, including MRSA, *E. coli* and *listeria*.

NOTE:

• Coriander seeds eaten in excess can have a narcotic effect.

Cumin *Cuminum cyminum*

References to cumin can be found in Sumerian and ancient Greek texts, and it was originally cultivated in Iran, around the Mediterranean and in the Nile valley. It should not be confused linguistically with *curcumin* (the French name for turmeric) or black cumin, or visually with caraway, which produces similar-looking seeds.

Cumin is one of the most widely used spices in the world, playing a significant role as a flavouring in many cuisines. The seeds are the dried fruits of a member of the parsley family (*Apiaceae*). The annual green plant grows to a height of about 30cm/12in, with a slender branched stem, thread-like leaves and white or pale pink small flowers set in umbels. The light brown seeds are tiny, ridged and often have a little stalk attached. Cumin needs a long, hot summer to mature to seed, and prefers full sun and a light, well-drained soil. It is now widely grown in India, the Middle East, North Africa, China and Mexico.

BUYING AND STORING

Buy dried seeds whole and store them in an airtight container out of direct sunlight. Toast the seeds just before using to bring out their full flavour. Once cool, grind them as required.

FOOD PROFILE

A staple of Asian cooking since ancient times, cumin is an essential flavouring in a wide range of curries and spice blends, and adds a warm, earthy flavour to cheeses, sauces, stews and soups. Cumin seeds have a distinctive, almost acrid scent and a strong, sharp flavour that is hot and aromatic, yet bitter. They are a key ingredient in many pickles, relishes and spice mixtures, including Harissa (see page 112).

NUTRITIONAL PROFILE

Cumin contains volatile oils, particularly cuminaldehyde, as well as flavonoids and phytoestrogens.

HEALTH PROFILE

Cumin is a traditional Indian remedy for digestive problems. It is also known to relieve cramps, to stimulate the flow of urine and to increase lactation. More recently, cumin seeds have been found to help reduce raised blood sugar and blood fats, and may thus slow the development of the complications of diabetes, such as cataracts. Cumin oil can be used externally to relieve swellings of the breasts and testicles.

NOTE:
- A tisane of 1 teaspoon of cumin seeds to 250ml/8fl oz/1 cup of boiling water, left to infuse for 10 minutes, makes a pleasant and beneficial digestive drink after meals.

Curry Leaf *Murraya koenigii*

The curry leaf, also known as sweet neem leaf or Indian bay, is native to South India and Sri Lanka, where it is still commonly found growing wild. It is also now grown in many other parts of the world, including Malaysia, Australia, South Africa and the West Indies, having been introduced by immigrants from the Indian subcontinent.

The curry tree belongs to the citrus family (*Rutaceae*) and can grow up to about 6m/20ft tall. The leaves consist of 11–21 narrow and highly aromatic small leaflets, each about 3cm/1¼in long. A mature tree can produce about 100kg/220lb of leaves per year. As the name suggests, fresh curry leaves have a distinct curry-like aroma when crushed and are a highly valued spice in Indian and Asian cuisine.

BUYING AND STORING

Fresh curry leaves can be bought in Asian food stores and markets, but can be hard to come by as they have a very short shelf life. Store them in a plastic bag in the refrigerator for about a week. It is possible to freeze fresh curry leaves, however, by leaving them on the stem and packing them in resealable freezer bags. They are also available dried, but the dried leaf has much less flavour than the fresh.

Alternatively, you can try growing your own curry tree in a container positioned in a hot and sheltered spot during summer and kept indoors at 12°C/54°F or above for the rest of the year. Pick fresh leaves directly from the stem as you need them.

FOOD PROFILE

Traditionally, fresh curry leaves are used in curry dishes, chopped together with onion and cooked gently in oil before adding the other ingredients. They can also be used in stir-fries, soups, pickles, chutneys, curry powders, dals and samosas.

NUTRITIONAL PROFILE

The curry leaf is rich in beta-carotene, vitamin C, folic acid, iron, calcium, phytosterols and carbazole alkaloids, and is reputed to have strong antioxidant properties.

HEALTH PROFILE

In Ayurvedic medicine, the curry leaf has long been used to reduce blood sugar, especially in the management of diabetes, and modern research has shown that curry leaves may help to slow the breakdown of starches and the uptake of glucose into the bloodstream. Consuming curry leaves may also help to lower blood cholesterol and blood fats.

Soap made from the volatile oil contained in the leaves has a wonderful lemony fragrance.

NOTE:

- Curry leaf is not the same as curry powder, and should not be confused with the garden curry plant, *Helichrysum italicum*.

Fennel Seed *Foeniculum vulgare*

Fennel is native to the Mediterranean coast but has become naturalized in many parts of the world, so much so that it is considered an invasive weed in parts of the United States and Australia. The fennel plant is a tall, hardy perennial member of the parsley family (*Apiaceae*). It can grow up to 2m/6ft high with hollow, ridged stems that carry aromatic feathery leaves and tiny bright yellow florets set in compound umbels of 20–50 flowers. The seeds are small, grooved, oblong and pale green with a distinctive, gentle aniseed fragrance and delicate flavour.

BUYING AND STORING

Fennel is widely cultivated and easy to grow as a garden plant. The seeds are ready to harvest when the umbels that contain them become pale green in colour. As fennel is closely related to dill, it can cross-fertilize, so it is best not to have these two plants near to each other.

Fennel seeds are available as a spice in most supermarkets, Asian food stores and health food stores. Always buy whole seeds as they soon lose their flavour once they are crushed or ground. Whole seeds stored in an airtight container away from direct sunlight will keep their flavour for several years.

FOOD PROFILE

Fennel has a long tradition as a seasoning for rich seafood dishes and sausages because it enhances their flavour and aids the digestion of fats. Very lightly toasted, crushed seeds impart a light, aniseedy taste to salad dressings and mayonnaise, and are often added to flavour breads, pancakes, cakes and cookies, and to make Indian-inspired soups, pickles, curries, dals and rice dishes.

Fennel seed is also one of the ingredients in a variety of spice mixes including Ras el Hanout (see page 110), Chinese Five Spice (see page 117) and Panch Phoron (see page 115). Indian restaurants often serve a mixed-seed dish known as a *mukhwa*, which includes fennel seeds, after a meal to aid digestion.

A tisane made from the seeds is a gentle after-dinner drink (see page 217). Take care not to make it too strong or leave it to infuse for too long as it then becomes unpleasant and bitter.

NUTRITIONAL PROFILE

Fennel seed contains volatile oils, including anethole, which provide the characteristic liquorice flavour. It also contains phytoestrogen, flavonoids, phytosterols and coumarins as well as linoleic, palmitic and oleic acid, which all show strong antioxidant activity.

HEALTH PROFILE

Fennel is a very effective digestive aid for easing stomach disorders and relieving wind and colic. It has a reputation for increasing milk flow and so can be a beneficial drink for nursing mothers. Its phytoestrogen content makes it a useful remedy for menstrual pain, and fennel is also a powerful antioxidant and anti-inflammatory, making it helpful in the management of chronic diseases such as arthritis. Fennel syrup is a traditional and effective cough remedy.

NOTES:
- Fennel seeds are sometimes confused with *Nigella sativa*, which is sometimes referred to as fennel flower, but nigella seeds are black and much smaller.

- Chewing fennel seeds can help to reduce the appetite and so some consider it an aid to slimming. They also freshen the breath.

Fenugreek Seed *Trigonella foenum-graecum*

Fenugreek is native to India and the Middle East, and archaeologists have found seeds in Iraq and Egypt that were dated at 4,000 years old. In the wild, fenugreek is found on sunny ground such as verges, dry grassland and hillsides.

The fenugreek plant is a green annual belonging to the legume family (*Fabaceae*). It grows up to 60cm/2ft high with small, clover-like leaves that are pale underneath, and pale yellow flowers. The amber-coloured seeds appear in long, narrow seedpods, each housing 10–20 seeds, which are easily recognizable by their triangular shape, with a deep groove running across one side, and their pungent aroma.

Fenugreek is also called bird's foot, Greek clover, *methi* and *hablah*. Its Latin name, *foenum-graecum,* translates as 'Greek hay' and the whole plant has long been grown for use as animal fodder. It is also applied as a natural fertilizer as it restores nitrogen to the soil. The seeds are popular both as a flavouring spice and a medicine.

BUYING AND STORING

Fenugreek is best bought as whole seeds, which can then be crushed or ground as required. The seeds will keep for up to 3 years in an airtight container stored out of direct sunlight.

FOOD PROFILE

Fenugreek seeds are commonly used to spice pickles, chutneys, curries, dals and curry powders. They have an aromatic, bittersweet flavour with a hint of celery, and are responsible for the distinctive smell of most commercially produced curry powders.

Raw fenugreek seeds taste bitter and astringent. Gently toasting the seeds in a hot pan before use enhances and sweetens their flavour and reduces their bitter taste. Toasted fenugreek seeds can be ground and used as a coffee substitute.

In India and the Middle East, fresh fenugreek leaves are eaten as a vegetable, often in combination with starchy root vegetables. The seeds are also easy to sprout and make delicious microgreens to add crunch and flavour to salads.

NUTRITIONAL PROFILE

Fenugreek seeds are high in protein and contain volatile oil, mucilage, alkaloids, saponins and plant sterols. An aromatic lactone called sotolone is responsible for the characteristic fenugreek aroma, a combination of curry and caramel.

HEALTH PROFILE

Fenugreek seeds can help to reduce blood sugar and may also reduce blood cholesterol levels. They are considered an aid to convalescence and are thought to help to improve milk flow in nursing mothers. They have a soothing effect on inflammation, which explains their traditional role in the treatment of stomach ulcers, colitis, diverticulitis and Crohn's disease. Externally, fenugreek seeds can be used to make a compress to relieve abscesses and swollen glands.

NOTE:

- 1–2 teaspoons of crushed seeds simmered in 250ml/8fl oz/1 cup of water for 15 minutes can be used as a skin lotion, or a conditioning rinse to nourish hair.

Galangal *Alpinia officinarum*

Galangal is native to China, where it is grown mainly on the southeast coast. It is also cultivated in India and other parts of Southeast Asia. Known variously as galanga, lesser galangal, galangale, colic root, Chinese ginger, *kencur* and East India Root, this spice comes from the dark reddish-brown fibrous rhizome of a member of the ginger family (*Zingiberaceae*). It looks like ginger and has an aromatic ginger-like scent, but it is much harder in texture and has a peppery, burnt, pungent taste. Like so many other traditional spices from the East, galangal is little known in the West today despite having been introduced to Europe by the Arabs long ago and used widely in the Middle Ages for its medicinal benefits.

BUYING AND STORING

Galangal root is available from Asian food stores, fresh, dried and sliced, or powdered. Store fresh galangal in the refrigerator for up to 2 weeks, or freeze flesh slices in a resealable plastic bag. Cut or powdered root should be stored in an airtight container, out of direct sunlight, and used within a year.

FOOD PROFILE

Galangal is widely used in Oriental cuisine (often in combination with garlic, ginger, chilli, lemon and tamarind), in fish and shellfish dishes and in sauces, soups, satays, sambals and curries. It also goes well in combination with fennel, lemongrass and coconut milk and is one of the essential ingredients in Thai curry pastes.

NUTRITIONAL PROFILE

Galangal contains galangol, kaempferol, cineol and linalol, as well as an acrid resin.

HEALTH PROFILE

Once described as the 'Spice of Life' by the medieval herbalist Hildegard of Bingen because of its stimulating properties, galangal aids digestion and metabolism and can relieve nausea, vomiting, sea-sickness, stomach ache, wind and indigestion. It also has a traditional role in the treatment of arthritis and diabetes, and as an antifungal remedy against *candida*.

NOTES:

- Polish vodka is often flavoured with galangal.
- To make a decoction, add ½ teaspoon of powdered galangal to 250ml/8fl oz/ 1 cup of water and simmer gently for 20 minutes. Drink 125ml/4fl oz/½ cup morning and evening.
- Galangal powder is sometimes taken as snuff.
- The name 'galangal' may also refer to two other ginger-family members popular in Asian cooking: greater galangal (*Alpinia galanga*) is less pungent and peppery, with orange/brown skin and pale yellow or white flesh. Aromatic ginger or sand ginger (*Kaempferia galanga*) has red skin, white flesh and a sweeter, almost sickly, pungent aroma and taste. This species is valued more for its medicinal properties than as a culinary flavouring.

Garlic *Allium sativum*

This strong-smelling, pungent-tasting bulb of the amaryllis family (*Amaryllidaceae*) is closely related to the onion, and has a history as a food and medicine going back more than 7,000 years. Even today, garlic products are top-selling supplements in pharmacies and health food stores, and fresh garlic is available in any store or market stall that sells vegetables. China is the world's leading garlic producer and exporter, cultivating more than 70% of the 17 million tonnes grown commercially in the world each year.

BUYING AND STORING

Fresh bulbs should be firm and closely packed, with creamy white or purple papery skin. Store in a cool, dry place out of direct sunlight.

FOOD PROFILE

Crushing, cutting or chopping garlic brings out its strong, sharp flavour. It is popular all over the world in dressings, sauces, pureés, marinades, butters, roasts, casseroles and stews. It is also delicious finely chopped into salads.

NUTRITIONAL PROFILE

Garlic has a high vitamin C and B6 content, and also contains vitamin B1, calcium, phosphorus, potassium, copper, manganese, selenium, antioxidant sulphur compounds, flavonoids and volatile oil containing high levels of allicin.

HEALTH PROFILE

Garlic has a proven reputation as an antibiotic active against bacteria, fungi and other infectious micro-organisms including *staphylococci*, *streptococci*, *E. coli*, *trichomonas*, *candida* and amoebic dysentery. It is a traditional remedy for treating colds, flu, bronchitis and asthma.

A growing body of scientific research confirms garlic's reputation for benefiting the cardiovascular system by lowering cholesterol, reducing blood clots (by preventing platelet aggregation), reducing atherosclerosis and lowering blood pressure.

Recently, it has been shown that garlic can help to lower blood glucose and thus reduce the risk of diabetes, and there is some evidence that eating garlic regularly may help prevent the development of an enlarged prostate in older men.

NOTES:
- To help remove the skin from a garlic clove, press down on it with the flat side of a large knife. Remove the skin, press again, sprinkle with a little salt, then chop.
- Eating fresh parsley with garlic helps to avoid bad garlic breath.

Ginger *Zingiber officinale*

Native to the tropical forests of Southeast Asia, ginger is now widely grown in Africa, Australia, Hawaii and the West Indies, but the world's biggest commercial producers are India and China.

Ginger has been valued as a spice and a medicine for over 3,000 years, and it was one of the first Oriental spices to be transported to the Mediterranean. It grows as a perennial subtropical plant of the ginger family (*Zingiberaceae*), with a rhizome that produces upright shoots that become leafy stems up to 1m/3ft tall. Yellow flowers appear in clusters from graceful pink and white flower buds, and when the stalks wither, the rhizome is harvested. Fresh ginger roots resemble deers' antlers, hence the Latin name *Zingiber*, which is thought to derive from the Sanskrit word *singabera*, meaning 'shaped like a horn'. The rhizomes of its close relatives galangal, turmeric and zedoary look very similar to root ginger.

BUYING AND STORING
Fresh ginger is available at most grocery stores, Asian stores and supermarkets. Choose plump, firm pieces that have smooth skin, wrap them in paper towels and store in the refrigerator for up to 3 weeks. Dried ginger slices are used traditionally for pickling, while ground ginger is used in baking and spice mixtures. Pickled ginger is served in Chinese and Japanese cuisine as a condiment, and crystallized/ candied ginger is popular as a snack, as confectionery or in desserts.

FOOD PROFILE
Fresh ginger adds a warm, woody-lemony flavour to cooked dishes and is an essential ingredient in curries and stir-fries. It can be used sliced, shredded,

chopped, grated or crushed, and makes an excellent addition to marinades and dressings. Root ginger is a key ingredient in many pickles, preserves, chutneys, cakes and breads.

NUTRITIONAL PROFILE

Raw ginger is rich in volatile oil and contains phenols, vitamins C and B6, magnesium, potassium and copper.

HEALTH PROFILE

For centuries, ginger has been taken to ease rheumatic complaints, and modern evidence confirms that it has an anti-inflammatory effect and may also lower blood pressure. It can aid slimming if taken as a hot drink with food because, as well as giving a sense of fullness, it enhances the thermic effect of food, reducing feelings of hunger. Widely used as a digestive aid, ginger can also be effective for motion sickness and nausea. It makes a warming drink and is thought to improve circulation.

NOTES:

- Start the day with a glass of hot water containing slices of lemon and ginger. Repeat with meals throughout the day.
- Use with caution during pregnancy. Ginger can be effective in treating morning sickness but avoid high doses and just before labour.

Horseradish *Armoracia rusticana*

Despite its name, horseradish is poisonous to horses. However, it is beneficial to people and has been used as a culinary and medicinal spice since ancient times. A member of the cabbage family (*Brassicaceae*), horseradish has been cultivated for centuries, mainly in Europe and North America, but also in parts of Australia, western Asia and the Middle East.

The horseradish is a perennial plant that grows up to 1m/3ft tall, produces large, long, wavy leaves, small white flowers and has long, white, fleshy roots. It grows best in light, moist soil and dappled shade or a sunny position.

The root, with its hot, fiery, mustard-like flavour, is valued as a spice, a medicine and a vegetable, raw or cooked. The young leaves can be eaten like spinach, raw or cooked, but be cautious as they do have a strong flavour. The root itself has little aroma until it is cut or grated, releasing tiny particles of mustard oil into the air.

BUYING AND STORING

Buy fresh roots and store, unwashed, in a plastic bag in the salad drawer/crisper of the refrigerator for several weeks, or store them in dry sand as this prevents them drying out and losing their flavour. Grate as required and use immediately, or add a little vinegar to prevent the flesh turning brown and bitter-tasting.

FOOD PROFILE

Though grated horseradish makes a delicious condiment on its own with a dash of vinegar, it is probably best known as an ingredient of horseradish sauce, made from grated horseradish, vinegar, salt, mustard and cream. Freshly grated horseradish mixed with cream and apples makes a refreshing side dish.

NUTRITIONAL PROFILE

Fresh horseradish contains vitamin C, volatile oils (including mustard oil), glycosides, peroxidase, coumarins, phenolic acids and resin.

HEALTH PROFILE

In traditional medicine, horseradish is used as an antifungal, antibacterial, urinary antiseptic, and as a pulmonary decongestant. New research also shows a promising effect on hyperthyroidism and on high blood cholesterol. As an external poultice, horseradish is often used to relieve sinusitis and joint and muscle pains. It is considered diuretic, stimulates skin, improves circulation and promotes sweating.

NOTES:

- To make a horseradish poultice, finely grate a fresh root, spread it on a thin cotton cloth and roll to make a pack. Place the pack on the skin and feel the heat. Remove when the warming heat turns into a burning sensation. If the skin is sensitive, rub a little petroleum jelly into the affected area before applying the poultice to avoid causing any further irritation.
- Remember that horseradish has a very strong flavour and contains mustard oil.

Consequently, it is better not to give it to young children or take during pregnancy, when breast-feeding, or by anyone suffering from gastrointestinal ulcers or kidney disease.

Jaggery *Saccharum officinarum*

Jaggery is a solid, unrefined sugar concentrate made from sugar cane, or from date, coconut or sago palm juice. Being unrefined, it is generally considered to be a healthier sweetener than other forms of sugar.

Originating from the Indian subcontinent, Sri Lanka and Africa, jaggery is also known as Burmese chocolate, medicinal sugar, *gur*, *gud* and *panela*. It is made by evaporating the raw cane juice or palm sap without separating the molasses from the crystals, and is boiled at 200°C/400°F in large, shallow, cast-iron vessels until it solidifies and becomes golden brown. It is available both as a paste and in blocks. The quality of jaggery is often judged by its colour: the more golden yellow being considered better quality than the darker products.

Used in Ayurvedic medicine for many centuries, jaggery is also a significant flavouring in sweet and savoury dishes. It has a religious role in Hinduism and it is considered advantageous to eat jaggery raw before embarking on any new work or venture. Jaggery is also shared to celebrate good news among family and friends.

BUYING AND STORING

Blocks of jaggery can be found in Indian grocery stores, Asian supermarkets, health food stores and online. It should be sticky and easy to crumble, rather than rock hard. Store it in an airtight container out of direct sunlight, and grate or crush it as required.

FOOD PROFILE

Richer in flavour than refined sugar, a little jaggery goes a long way in the kitchen. It is, of course, high in calories but as less is required for flavour, it is often better tolerated than refined sugar. Jaggery can be used to sweeten savoury dishes, to lessen the acidity of tomatoes and to balance the spicy, salty, sweet and sour flavours of a dish. Popularly used in sambals, it is also great in desserts, cakes, confectionery, chutneys, creams and drinks, and can be used to make alcoholic beverages.

NUTRITIONAL PROFILE

Being unrefined and prepared in cast-iron vessels, jaggery contains iron and trace minerals and vitamins, including vitamin B2, calcium, iron, magnesium, phosphorus, potassium, zinc, copper and manganese.

HEALTH PROFILE

In Ayurvedic medicine, jaggery is called *guda* and is mentioned in texts dating back 2,500 years. It has been used traditionally to ease digestion and relieve constipation, and to reduce anaemia, relieve headaches and to treat coughs and colds. It is also applied in body scrubs.

NOTES:

- Make Panakam juice (a cooling drink for sipping in very hot weather) by dissolving a little jaggery in hot water, and mixing in a shake of black pepper and a little crushed cardamom. Serve chilled.
- Create a nourishing and revitalizing body scrub by mixing equal quantities of jaggery and coconut oil. Use immediately or store in an airtight container for up to 1 week.
- Light muscovado/brown sugar makes a good alternative to jaggery in recipes, although it lacks the distinctive caramel flavour.

Juniper *Juniperus communis*

Juniper is one of the few spices that grows in a cool, temperate climate. It is distributed throughout the Northern Hemisphere, from the Arctic to Africa, Europe, Asia and the mountains of North and Central America. It is a species of coniferous shrub belonging to the cypress family (*Cupressaceae*) that is commonly found as a low-spreading dense, scrub bush, which has sharp, needle-like leaves and grows best in dry conditions. The species is extremely old and has been utilized as a fuel, medicine, preservative and flavouring since ancient times.

Juniper berries are tiny conifer cones with fleshy scales that merge to contain the seeds. The green berries take 18 months or more to ripen, turning dark purple with a blue waxy tint. The berries on the same bush don't all ripen simultaneously and only fully ripe ones should be used.

BUYING AND STORING

Dried juniper berries are available in supermarkets and health food stores, and should be kept whole in an airtight container out of direct sunlight. Even when dried, they are slightly soft and easy to crush. They can last several years but must be discarded if any show signs of mould.

FOOD PROFILE

Eating a fresh juniper berry direct from the bush gives a clear indication of its botanical origin: it tastes of pine resin and turpentine with a bittersweet, tart note that is not unpleasant, but enjoyed more by birds and wildlife than people. When dried, crushed and used sparingly in food and drink, however, juniper berries can enhance and bring out the best in other flavours.

Traditionally used as the flavouring for gin, juniper berries also go well with fruits, especially in cakes, and also in rich stews, pâtés, pickles and marinades. Juniper berries are very popular in the Nordic kitchen where they are often used to flavour herring, cabbage dishes, including sauerkraut, and beer.

NUTRITIONAL PROFILE

Juniper berries contain tannins, sugars, resin, bitter principle (juniperine) and volatile oils (including pinene, borneol, cadinene, camphene, terpenic alcohol and terpineol).

HEALTH PROFILE

Juniper berries are a strong urinary tract antiseptic and diuretic, and have been used traditionally to reduce oedema, treat bladder stones and reduce inflammation in cases of gout and arthritis. The berries can be eaten or made into a tisane, but take no more than 15 berries per day, and take for short periods of time only. Juniper is also a traditional ingredient in aperitifs, such as Martini, that help to stimulate appetite and aid digestion. Applied externally in bathwater, juniper can treat skin problems, colds and painful joints, and is also added to perfume toiletries and deodorants. It is also considered effective as an insect repellent on exposed wounds.

NOTES:

- Juniper berries have an old reputation as a natural contraceptive and so should be avoided in pregnancy.
- Large doses can cause damage to the kidneys, so juniper should not be used therapeutically by anyone with kidney disease.

Kaffir Lime *Citrus hystrix*

Also known as Mauritius papeda, *magrood, makrut* and Thai lime, kaffir lime is a highly aromatic but thorny tropical bush belonging to the citrus family (*Rutaceae*). Native to Southeast Asia, the plant is cultivated throughout the region and provides some of the essential flavourings used in Indonesian, Vietnamese and Thai cuisines.

The shrub grows 5–10m/16–32ft tall and produces distinct, fragrant double leaves that look as if one leaf is growing on the end of another. It has attractive waxy flowers and produces small, intricately wrinkled, bright green fruits that are bitter and full of pips.

The kaffir lime is also a popular garden shrub, well suited to patio containers and conservatories. It is easy to grow but requires protection from the cold, needing a temperature of at least 12–15°C/53–59°F to thrive. The leaves and fruits are valued in the preparation of food, drinks and medicines.

BUYING AND STORING

For the best flavour, buy fresh leaves whenever possible. They are available at Asian food stores, often frozen and do not need thawing. Dried kaffir lime leaves are more commonplace but are less fragrant. Look for green leaves, not yellow. Stored in an airtight container away from heat, sun and humidity, they should last for up to a year.

Kaffir lime fruits can be difficult to find fresh, but they freeze well, too, and the zest can be grated directly off the frozen fruit.

FOOD PROFILE

In Southeast Asian cuisines, the leaves are the most commonly used part of the plant. They impart that characteristic fragrant, lemony taste to Thai, Indonesian, Balinese,

Javanese, Cambodian and Vietnamese curries, and can add an extra fresh, almost floral flavour to steamed vegetables, rice dishes, soups, salads and stir-fries.

Prepare fresh or frozen leaves by cutting or shredding them finely and removing the tough midrib. If you use dried leaves they should be removed before serving.

The zest of the bitter fruit is added to curry pastes and marries particularly well with dishes containing coconut cream, fish, chicken and strong spices. In Creole cuisine, the rind is used to flavour rums, and in Cambodia, kaffir limes are candied whole as a sweet delicacy. The juice from the kaffir lime is very pungent and bitter so should be used sparingly.

NUTRITIONAL PROFILE

The essential oil, found mainly in the leaves and in the fruit rind, is responsible for the kaffir lime's beautiful lemony scent and flavour. It contains citronellol, citronellal, nerol and limonene. Some of these constituents are also found in citronella, lemon balm and lemongrass, which also have insect repellent properties.

HEALTH PROFILE

Chewing kaffir lime leaves, rubbing them on your gums or using the essential oil in toothpastes is recommended for promoting healthy gums and white teeth.

The volatile oil is recognized as a strong insect repellent and is used in ointments and sprays, as well as in deodorants, hair conditioners, soaps and shampoos. Besides being considered a fine hair and scalp cleanser, kaffir lime juice and its aromatic properties are also reputed to have a rejuvenating effect on the mind, easing away negative thoughts and evil spirits.

On the more practical side, the astringent juice can act as a natural bleach and may remove stains from some fabrics.

NOTES:
- If kaffir lime is not available, lemongrass or ordinary lime peel can be used as a substitute in recipes.
- Halve a kaffir lime and rub it in your hair and scalp after shampooing instead of using conditioner.

Kokum *Garcinia indica*

Also known as *aamsul* or sour apple, the kokum tree is a fruit-bearing evergreen belonging to the mangosteen family (*Clusiaceae*) and grows widely in Indian rainforests. It can reach a height of 20m/65ft and prefers a hot and humid climate. The kokum tree takes about 10 years of growth before it starts bearing fruits, which in turn take many months to ripen. The ripe fruits turn deep purple after harvesting and keep for only about five days. They are tasty with a sweet yet sour and distinctly cooling flavour.

Ripe kokum are halved and dried out in the sun, and may also be smoked. The dried outer skin is the spice, and the dried seeds, which are rich in oil and the source of kokum butter, are also used in the manufacture of confectionery and cosmetics.

BUYING AND STORING

Dried kokum is dark purple or black, resembling a thick plum. It will keep for about a year in an airtight container out of direct sunlight. It is available at Asian food stores and markets.

FOOD PROFILE

Kokum adds a pink or purple colour and a sweet-sour taste to foods, and is used to flavour curries, chutneys and soups; in cooling syrups and drinks; and as a garnish. Like tamarind, it should be infused in hot water before use, and the quality of the spice is indicated by the intensity of the colour of the resultant purple-pink liquid.

NUTRITIONAL PROFILE

Kokum contains anthocyanin pigments, tannins, pectin, omega oils, hydroxycitric acid (HCA), garcinol, citric acid, oxalic acid and ascorbic acid. HCA may promote body fat loss, and is known to suppress appetite. Garcinol is attracting interest as a potent antioxidant, anti-cancer and antiviral agent.

HEALTH PROFILE

A kokum infusion can be taken as a drink, or applied directly to skin rashes, burns and dry skin for its cooling effect. It is used traditionally to treat intestinal worms, dysentery, indigestion, piles and heart conditions, and kokum syrup is considered helpful in treating sunstroke. Kokum butter is soothing and astringent and is used in ointments, suppositories and other pharmaceutical products designed to treat ulcers, fissures and cracked skin.

NOTE:
- 3–4 dried kokum halves are enough to flavour most dishes.

Lemongrass *Cymbopogon citratus*

Also known as camel's hay, citronella, silky heads, fever grass and *hierba luisa*, lemongrass is a tall, perennial, tropical grass with a solid, bulbous white base that resembles a small, pale spring onion/scallion. A member of the true grass family (*Gramineae*), it prefers dense turfs and a tropical or subtropical climate. Lemongrass is grown throughout southern India, Sri Lanka, Southeast Asia, the West Indies, Brazil, Guatemala, Mexico and Central Africa.

The plant's stems, leaves and base smell of fresh lemons and can be used to add a vibrant citrus flavour, with a hint of ginger, to many dishes. Only the lower end of the stem is sliced into rings for cooking. Lemongrass oil is a natural preservative and insect repellent, which nevertheless attracts bees.

A close cousin, citronella grass, is distinguished by its red stem base, and provides citronella oil, an insect repellent used in sprays, soaps and candles.

BUYING AND STORING
Bunches of fresh lemongrass stalks are sold in supermarkets and Asian food stores, and the spice is also available as a dried ground powder called *sereh*: 1 teaspoon of powder is roughly equivalent to one fresh stalk. Dried lemongrass slices are also available and should be soaked for 2 hours before use. Fresh lemongrass offers the best flavour and, if wrapped in a paper bag, will keep for a week or so in the salad drawer/crisper of a refrigerator. It can also be frozen and defrosted as required.

FOOD PROFILE
Whole stalks, or slices from the lower stem and bulb, are used in a wide variety of

savoury dishes, pickles and marinades to give a gentle and refreshing hint of lemon.

Lemongrass is fibrous and unpleasant to eat so the stalks should be bashed just before cooking to release their flavour, then removed before serving. Alternatively, cut off the root end of the stalk, remove the tough outer leaves, then slice the stem from the base up until you no longer see a purple band in the flesh. Or you can simply pound the stalks with other ingredients to form a paste.

Lemongrass combines particularly well with coconut milk, garlic, shallots, chillies and coriander/cilantro leaves.

NUTRITIONAL PROFILE
Scientific analysis shows that lemongrass contains a number of phytochemicals, notably citral and various phytosterols.

HEALTH PROFILE
Lemongrass has marked antifungal, antibacterial, anti-inflammatory and diuretic properties, and is used traditionally to treat sore throats, fevers and infections, including thrush. Research has also shown that lemongrass may inhibit cancer cell growth, lower cholesterol and help control type-2 diabetes. It has a soothing, sedating effect, useful in cases of anxiety and insomnia, and it also induces sweating, which may explain its role in the management of fever.

NOTES:
- Try a refreshing lemongrass tisane (*chukku kappi*) made with slices of fresh or frozen stem base in boiling water.
- If you find a fresh lemongrass stalk with some root still attached, you can try and grow lemongrass as a houseplant. Put the stalk in a jar of water and more roots should soon develop. Once a number of roots have grown, pot the plant into some potting compost/soil and it should flourish.

Mace 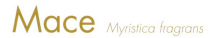 *Myristica fragrans*

Mace is the bright red outer shell, or aril, of the nut-like seed of the nutmeg tree, an evergreen tree of the nutmeg family (*Myristicaceae*)(see pages 70–71).

Nutmeg trees take 7–9 years to mature and bear fruit, and at least another 10 years before they become fully productive. The lacy, bright red mace turns more orangey-yellow after it is broken off the nutmeg in pieces known as blades.

For centuries, the Banda Islands in the Moluccas (once known as the Spice Islands) of Indonesia were the only place where the nutmeg tree would grow. Today it is cultivated in Sri Lanka, India, Malaysia and the West Indies, notably Grenada, as well as Indonesia.

The slow-growing nutmeg tree is the only tree to produce two different spices from one nut, and the fact that it could only be grown on a few remote islands once made mace, along with nutmeg, one of the rarest and most valued spices. Even today, mace has a higher commercial value than nutmeg because it is far more scarce: 10kg/22lb of nutmegs provides only 100g/3½oz of mace.

BUYING AND STORING

Mace is sold either in blades or ground to a brown, orange-tinted powder. The best-quality blades are slightly bendy and release a little oil when squeezed, but dried blades can be hard to crush and should be soaked in a little water before use, then removed after cooking.

FOOD PROFILE

Mace and nutmeg have similar qualities, but mace is considered both the more delicate and the more powerful of the two spices. It has a sweet, fragrant aroma, and a mild, warm, intense, sweet-sharp flavour. It adds colour and a mild nutmeg flavour to soups and sauces, sausages, pâtés and potato dishes, and gives a fine hint of burnt orange to milky and creamy dishes, cakes and mashed potatoes. A little mace added to chocolate drinks and tropical fruit juices also helps to bring out and round off their full flavours.

NUTRITIONAL PROFILE

Mace contains volatile oil, gum, resin and fixed oils.

HEALTH PROFILE

Mace can be used to stimulate appetite, aid digestion, relieve colic and wind, and treat intestinal infections. Excessive use may produce a mild narcotic effect and could also cause overexcitement.

Mahlab *Prunus mahaleb*

Also known as mahlap, mahalep and mahlepi, mahlab is an aromatic spice made from the seed kernels of the mahaleb cherry tree (also known as the St Lucie cherry or rock cherry tree). It is a member of the rose family (*Rosaceae*) and can be found growing wild on dry hillsides, in thickets and in open woodland throughout central and southern Europe. Commercial production of mahlab is concentrated in Iran, Turkey and Syria, although it is also grown as an ornamental tree in Europe and the US.

The cherries are small, slightly oval, green fruits that turn black when ripe. The small cherry pits are cracked open to extract their pale tan seeds, the mahlab. These are ground to a creamy-yellow powder, which is popular in baked products and pastries, especially in Arab, Turkish, Greek and Armenian cuisines.

BUYING AND STORING

Look out for mahlab seeds in Middle Eastern grocery stores, especially around Easter time. Always buy them whole and grind only as required because they soon lose their intensity, aroma and flavour once ground, and the powder tends to turn rancid after a short time. Store the whole seeds in an airtight container in a cool place, away from direct sunlight.

FOOD PROFILE

Mahlab seeds have a distinct, bittersweet, almond-cherry flavour with a hint of marzipan and a slightly bitter aftertaste. Used in small quantities (I recommend a maximum of 1 teaspoon per 500g/1lb 2oz/4 cups of flour), they give a characteristic Middle Eastern flavour to breads, cookies, cakes, pastries, desserts and snacks.

NUTRITIONAL PROFILE

Mahlab contains fixed oil, fatty acids, coumarins and sugars.

HEALTH PROFILE

Mahlab is a gentle remedy that has a tonic effect on the digestive system and a calming effect on the nerves, producing a feeling of general wellbeing. It has been applied in the treatment of asthma and also as an antibacterial remedy against enterobacteria. Mahlab is thought to have anti-diabetic and diuretic properties.

NOTES:

- Mahlab seeds should only be used in small amounts. Very bitter seeds should not be eaten as they contain the poison hydrogen cyanide (the same chemical that is found in bitter almonds).
- Grind the seeds with sugar or salt crystals to help make a powder.

Melegueta Pepper *Aframomum melegueta*

Native to the coastal swamps of West Africa from Sierra Leone to the Congo, melegueta pepper is also known as grains of paradise, Guinea grains, Guinea pepper, alligator pepper and *fom wisa*. The tiny reddish-brown, grain-like seeds are obtained from the dried fruits of a herbaceous perennial and member of the ginger family (*Zingiberaceae*). Imported into Europe along the spice routes through the Sahara desert, melegueta pepper was a more affordable substitute for the much more expensive black pepper, particularly during the 14th and 15th centuries, before the introduction of the *capsicum* species to Europe. For centuries, melegueta was used by herbalists to stimulate circulation and the immune system, and it was held in such high esteem as a spice that its native habitat was named the Grain Coast in its honour.

Melegueta fruits can be eaten fresh and their seeds have an aromatic, pungent, peppery taste with a hint of ginger and nutmeg. These can be used like cardamom or black pepper, crushed in a mortar, grinder or pepper mill. Toast first to bring out their full flavour.

Melegueta was a popular spice and a medicine in Great Britain until the 19th century, when King George III forbade its use on grounds of it giving 'fictitious strength' to cordials and aquavits. After that, its importation dropped off rapidly and soon it was largely forgotten and replaced by other fiery spices and peppers.

BUYING AND STORING

Melegueta pepper is available in speciality culinary stores and markets. Whole grains stored in an airtight container, out of direct sunlight, should keep their flavour for up to 4 years.

FOOD PROFILE

Melegueta pepper adds a fantastically pungent and hot peppery taste to savoury dishes, raw foods, bakes and desserts. It also adds a spicy flavour to gins, vinegars, Scandinavian akvavits and beers. A favourite spice in West African cookery, melegueta is currently enjoying renewed popularity after being rediscovered by celebrity chefs. It can be beneficial in raw food diets as it is less of an irritant to the digestive system than black pepper.

NUTRITIONAL PROFILE

Melegueta pepper contains volatile oils, saponins, glycosides, flavonoids, and phyto-sterols.

HEALTH PROFILE

Melegueta pepper is a powerful antioxidant and contains volatile oils, alkaloids, glycosides, tannins, flavonoids and phytosterols. It has anti-inflammatory, antimicrobial and antifungal properties, and a warming and stimulating effect on digestion and circulation. It also appears to have some anti-diabetic and body-fat-reducing properties, and has a reputation as an aphrodisiac.

NOTE:

- As with many other hot spices, large amounts of melegueta pepper should be avoided in pregnancy.

MUSTARD SEED *Brassica juncea, B. nigra and Sinapis alba*

Mustards are part of the cabbage family (*Brassicaceae*). Many well-known food plants (for example, cabbages, kale, cauliflower, broccoli, turnips and radishes) are from the same genus, and the old family name refers to the four-petalled flowers characteristic of this plant group. Black mustard is thought to originate from the

Mediterranean region and was used in ancient Greece. White mustard is native to Europe and yellow mustard is believed to originate in central Asia.

Mustard prefers light, moist, well-drained soil and a sunny or semi-shaded position. It is an annual green plant with small yellow flowers that appear through the summer and go to seed in early autumn/fall. Mustard seeds are small, round and hard; coloured pale beige, brown or black; with no aroma, although the leaves and flowers smell faintly of mustard. The leaves and stems are delicious eaten as a vegetable, raw, steamed and stir-fried, and can even be pickled.

Mustard plants are also grown and applied as a green manure and for mulching. They have a special ability to absorb micronutrients and tolerate heavy metals, which makes them useful for removing contaminants from the soil in an elegant and inexpensive way.

An unusual fact about the term 'mustard' is that the name of the condiment gave name to the plant, rather than vice versa: it derives from the ancient Roman flavouring made by grinding mustard seeds and mixing them with *mustum* (Latin for unfermented grape juice) to make a paste known as *mustum ardens* (burning paste).

BUYING AND STORING

White mustard seeds are light beige in colour, have a mild flavour and are ground to make powdered mustard and for pickling. Yellow mustard seeds are smaller than white and vary in colour from light to dark brown. They are often used in the making of curry powders and pastes. Black mustard seeds are small, dark brown to black grains and the most pungent and fiery of the mustard family. They are used in Indian cooking, toasted in hot oil or ghee, and to make Bordeaux mustard. Black mustard is easy to grow, but is hard to harvest mechanically and so can be less readily available commercially.

Whole mustard seeds will keep for more than a year if stored out of direct sunlight in an airtight container. Prepared mustard can last for at least a year if kept in a sealed jar in the refrigerator. The sign of a mustard blend being past its best is when the liquid separates from the solids, which then become thicker and darker. Mustard powder generally has a long shelf life of about 2 years, but loses its potency over time.

FOOD PROFILE

In medieval Europe, mustard was the only affordable spice commonly available to ordinary people for adding extra flavour to their bland food. With the gradual introduction of an expanding range of exotic spices from the 16th century onward, mustard lost some of its ubiquity. However, it is still a significant spice in most kitchens as it is the key ingredient in one of our most popular condiments, with an annual world consumption of well over 200 million kilos/440 million pounds.

Whole mustard seeds can be used raw, sprouted or toasted, and are widely used in pickling spices, partly for their flavour and partly for their preservative qualities.

White mustard seeds are ground and made into mustard powder, which tastes bland until mixed with cold water. An enzyme in the powder then facilitates a chemical reaction that brings out the full flavour in about 10 minutes. Both hot water and vinegar block this reaction, and so should not be used to make mustard paste (though they can, of course, be added later).

All three types of mustard seed can be used whole, toasted or ground with other spices for flavouring sauces, baked beans and many other dishes. They also add flavour and punch when sprinkled on salads and raw foods.

NUTRITIONAL PROFILE

Mustard contains volatile oil, omega oils, protein, carbohydrate, fibre, sterols, enzymes, allyl isothiocyanate, glucosinolates, mucilage and erucic acid.

HEALTH PROFILE

In herbal medicine, mustard seeds are used to make external poultices to stimulate circulation and relieve muscle or joint pain. A mustard poultice applied to the chest is also effective for relieving coughs and breathlessness in chronic obstructive pulmonary disease (COPD).

Internally, mustard seeds have a traditional reputation for their warming quality, and their mildly irritant effect may be useful in the treatment of fevers, colds, sinusitis, bronchitis and influenza. In recent research, mustard seed oil has been shown to reduce blood cholesterol levels and may have the potential to lower the risk of cardiovascular disease and slow the development of cancer cells when eaten daily as part of a healthy diet.

NOTES:

- To make a mustard poultice, mix freshly ground seeds with a little lukewarm water to form a thick paste. Spread the paste on a piece of cotton material to form a pack. Lay the pack on the affected area and then remove after 1 minute. Rub the skin gently with sweet almond oil afterwards.

- To make a warming mustard infusion, use 1 teaspoon of ground seeds to 250ml/ 8fl oz/1 cup of boiling water and leave to infuse for 5 minutes.
- Chilblains can be relieved with a hand or foot bath containing 1 tablespoon of ground mustard seeds.

WARNING:

- Be aware that mustard can be an irritant to sensitive skins.

NIGELLA SEEDS *Nigella sativa*

Also known as black cumin, *kalonji*, blessed seed, blackseed, black caraway, onion seed and black sesame, nigella is native to Asia and the Middle East, and most widely cultivated in India. Its seeds can be traced back through biblical times to ancient Egypt and the tomb of Tutankhamun. Over the centuries, nigella seeds have been used by herbalists and healers as a cure-all but, until recently, interest in their medicinal properties had waned in the West as non-medicinal cultivars (such as *Nigella damascena*) were developed and grew in popularity as decorative garden plants.

Nigella sativa (also known variously as Roman coriander, nutmeg flower and fennel flower) is a member of the buttercup family (*Ranunculaceae*) and a self-seeding herbaceous annual, growing up to 60cm/2ft tall. In the summer, nigella produces delicate white flowers that have faint blue- or green-tinted petal tips. These are followed by seedpods that are large, oblong, decorative capsules with up to seven follicles (compartments) containing rows of tightly packed seeds.

BUYING AND STORING

Nigella seeds are small, fat and triangular with a deep matte-black colour, a pleasantly bitter, peppery taste and a noticeably crunchy texture. Confusingly, the name 'black cumin' (by which nigella seeds are sometimes known) is also applied to another spice, *Bunium persicum* (see page 25), and the two are often confused in recipes. They are quite different in taste, texture and appearance, however: *Bunium persicum* is closely related to caraway and cumin (from the *Apiaceae* family) and has long, narrow ridged seeds, darker than ordinary cumin but not the deep black of nigella. Nigella seeds are available in Asian food stores, and can be used whole, crushed or ground. Stored in an airtight container, out of direct sunlight, they will last for several years.

FOOD PROFILE

Nigella is probably best recognized as the tiny black seeds sprinkled on Turkish bread and Indian naan. Nigella seeds are also popular in many parts of the world for adding flavour to cheeses, chutneys, stews, pilafs, confectionery and liqueurs, and are sometimes enjoyed as a condiment in place of black pepper.

NUTRITIONAL PROFILE

Nigella seeds are high in protein (21%), rich in polyunsaturated oils (up to 35%) and important omega oils, particularly linoleic acid, which nourish the immune system and protect the heart.

HEALTH PROFILE

Modern research has confirmed the traditional view of nigella as a healer for a wide range of chronic health problems, including cardiovascular disorders, allergies and cancer. The hint of thyme in the seeds' flavour comes from the phytochemical thymoquinone, a powerful antioxidant, and consuming nigella seeds on a regular basis has been proven to boost the action of the immune system. This, together with their marked anti-inflammatory action, also makes nigella seeds effective in the relief of allergic reactions such as hayfever, asthma and eczema, and some food companies have filed patent applications for the use of nigella seeds in the treatment of allergies.

Nigella has been shown to improve lung function by dilating the airways, and can thus be of use in the treatment of bronchitis and various other respiratory problems. If the seeds, or seed extract, are used regularly, they also have a beneficial effect on the heart and circulation by gently lowering blood pressure and circulating cholesterol levels. Nigella's ability to stop cells mutating suggests that it may have a role in cancer management, where slowing the rate of tumour cell division is one of the primary aims. Other studies have reported positive results when using nigella seeds to treat stomach ulcers and colitis, as well as degenerative conditions such as multiple sclerosis and neurological disorders including epilepsy.

NOTES:

- Nigella is one of the five spices included in Panch Phoron (see page 115), also known as Bengali five spice.
- Toasting nigella seeds in a hot frying pan just before use brings out their full flavour and makes them easier to grind.

NUTMEG *Myristica fragrans*

Nutmeg is the seed of the fruit of the nutmeg tree, one of the nutmeg family (*Myristicaceae*). The tree is tropical and evergreen, and can grow up to 20m/66ft tall. Native to the Banda Islands in the Moluccas (one of the group once known as the Spice Islands), Indonesia, the nutmeg tree prefers a hot and humid climate, and is now grown commercially in Indonesia and the West Indies, notably Grenada, and also in Sri Lanka, Malaysia, India and Papua New Guinea.

It takes 6–8 years before the female trees flower and produce fruit (the male trees are unproductive), but there is no way of distinguishing a female tree from a male until they start flowering. Nutmeg trees reach full maturity after 15–20 years and can carry on producing fruit for another 50 years or more. A fully mature tree can produce more than 2,000 nutmegs per year.

The fruit of the nutmeg tree is a pale yellow edible drupe that resembles an apricot. When ripe, it splits to expel the seed, which is covered in a hard shell surrounded by a bright red lace covering, called the aril. This net-like aril is called mace (see page 61), and the hard, small, slightly wrinkled, egg-shaped seed inside is the nutmeg. Nutmegs and mace are dried separately when the fruit is harvested.

Mentioned by Pliny back in the 1st century and used in Roman times to fumigate houses, nutmeg had reached Byzantium by the 6th century and has been used as a medicine ever since. The Persian doctor, Ibn Sina, wrote about the 'Banda nut' about 300 years later and nutmeg was first imported to Europe by the Arabs. It became very fashionable, especially among the wealthy, and was central to the economics of the spice trade for hundreds of years. In the 16th century, the Portuguese claimed the Banda Islands and thus took control of the valuable and prized nutmeg trade. In the 17th century, it shared the same fate as cloves in the battle for spice-trade supremacy between the Portuguese and the Dutch (see pages 37–38), and again it was Pierre Poivre, the bold French horticulturalist, who managed to smuggle nutmegs and cloves out of the East Indies and start a plantation on the island of Mauritius. By the end of the 18th century, the British had taken control of the Spice Islands and spread cultivation of nutmeg to their other colonies. Today, nutmeg is produced in Indonesia, Malaysia, India and the Caribbean island of Grenada, where the nutmeg has become so significant to the economy that it now calls itself 'Nutmeg Island' and features a nutmeg on its flag.

BUYING AND STORING

Nutmeg is available as a ground spice, but is best bought whole to be grated as required (dainty nutmeg graters are often sold alongside the nuts). One whole nutmeg grated yields 2–3 teaspoons of powder, but the taste is very intense so only a pinch is needed. Whole nutmegs will keep for years stored in an airtight jar out of direct sunlight.

FOOD PROFILE

Nutmeg and mace have similar qualities, but nutmeg has a stronger, slightly sweeter, more pungent flavour. The taste and scent is warm, aromatic and nutty, and goes well with sweet and spicy drinks and dishes. Nutmeg is a popular ingredient in spice blends, notably garam masala, and has a particular ability to balance the richness of foods it is added to. A little nutmeg enhances the flavour of potato and tomato dishes, and is delicious sprinkled on steamed or raw vegetables. It is also added to many processed foods to enhance the flavour, and is found in many recipes for soups, white sauces, casseroles, curries and pasta dishes, and in cocktails, ciders, mulled wines and eggnog.

NUTRITIONAL PROFILE

Nutmeg contains about 10% volatile oil, including camphene, pinene, thujene, linalool, terpineol, myristicin and eugenol among others. It also contains fixed oils and phenolic compounds.

HEALTH PROFILE

In the Middle Ages, nutmeg was highly prized and believed to have magical powers. People even carried nutmeg around with them in a small locket on a chain, accompanied by a special grater made of wood, ivory or silver. It was said to comfort the head and the nerves, and was known to calm the digestion while stimulating the circulation. In small quantities, nutmeg was administered as a sedative and given to children (grated with food or as a tisane) to relieve indigestion, colic, nausea, vomiting, wind and diarrhoea.

Modern research has shown nutmeg to be among the strongest antioxidants and an effective antibacterial and anti-inflammatory plant medicine able to increase calmness while reducing feelings of anger and embarrassment. It has also been found to inhibit blood clotting and to decrease prostaglandin levels in the colon, making it useful in the management of Crohn's disease. Extracts of nutmeg inhibit leukaemia cell development, and compounds within it have been found to inhibit the breakdown of elastin in the skin and thus keep the skin more supple.

Nutmeg contains sufficient fixed oils to make nutmeg butter, which is used in some beauty and skin products. Nutmeg also seems to help protect the skin from over-exposure to harmful UV sun-rays.

However, nutmeg does have a reputation as an intoxicant that can cause hallucinations and euphoria, together with palpitations, nausea, headache, dizziness, dry mouth and delirium, but the psychoactive effect is only seen in large doses and varies markedly from person to person. Nutmeg intoxication may last for several hours (and the side effects for several days), and is caused mainly by myristicin poisoning, which is potentially fatal for pets and livestock.

NOTES:
- To relieve joint pain, try an ointment made by mixing freshly grated nutmeg, ginger, ground cloves and citronella oil with ground, uncooked rice. Apply to the affected joint and leave to soak into the skin.
- Grated nutmeg mixed with coconut oil is a traditional external remedy for haemorrhoids.
- Nutmeg is not related to nuts, and does not normally provoke an allergic reaction.

WARNING:
- As mentioned above, large doses of nutmeg are toxic and can cause hallucinations and palpitations. As it was once used in large doses to provoke abortion, nutmeg should be used with care during pregnancy.

Paprika *Capsicum annuum*

Paprika is made from the dried fruit pods of the sweet capsicum, an annual, densely branched shrub that is a member of the nightshade family (*Solanaceae*). The plant has dark green leaves and single white flowers that develop into green pepper fruits. The peppers turn red, purple or brown as they ripen, ready for harvesting at the end of the summer. There are many different varieties of capsicum (see pages 32–34), but only the red fruits are used to make paprika.

As a tropical plant native to South America, sweet capsicum was introduced into Europe by Spanish and Portuguese explorers in the 16th century. Eventually it has become acclimatized to cooler climates, and is now grown commercially in Hungary and Spain, and also in North and South America, Morocco, Turkey and central Europe. Although different varieties of paprika vary from mild and sweet to hot and pungent, they are all much milder, warmer and sweeter than the original tropical capsicum fruits from which they are descended.

Hungarian paprika is bright red and has a characteristic rich flavour. It is graded from delicate (Kulonleges) to hot and pungent (Eros), with four grades in between. Hungarian paprika is often specified in recipes because of its unique flavour. Spanish paprika is sweeter and milder, with varieties ranging from sweet (*pimentón dulce*) via semi-sweet (*pimentón agridulce*) to hot (*pimentón picante*). Smoked paprika is made by slow-oak-smoking three different types of pepper, sweet, bittersweet and hot, which are ground together to a fine powder. Hungarian rose paprika, made from only the choicest fruits, is highly prized for its brilliant colour and sweet aroma.

BUYING AND STORING

Paprika is only available ready-ground, so buy it in small quantities and store in an airtight container out of direct sunlight.

FOOD PROFILE

Paprika is used commercially in snack and convenience foods, as well as in a wide range of dishes including tomato sauces, cheeses, soups, processed foods and as a food colouring (listed as 'natural colour' on the label). The flavour varies depending on the kind of paprika used, but it is never as spicy as cayenne pepper or chilli powder. Its main purpose is to add flavour and colour rather than heat. Paprika is best known as the principal spice in Hungarian goulash, but is also widely used in many other national cuisines, including Spanish, Portuguese, Austrian, Greek, Turkish, Croatian and Moroccan.

NUTRITIONAL PROFILE

Paprika is very high in vitamin A, as well as vitamins C, E, B2, B3, B6 and iron, capsaicin, carotenoids and fibre.

HEALTH PROFILE

Anti-inflammatory and antioxidant, paprika is an excellent source of carotenoids, which can benefit the immune system.

NOTES:

- Some people like to add a spoonful of paprika to henna hair dye to give an extra-red tint.
- For maximum flavour impact, paprika should be added to hot oil to dissolve the powder and help release the aroma. It is important to be careful, however, because the spice turns bitter and unpleasant if burnt. For best results, add to a pan or to a stew when piping hot and then reduce to a simmer.

PEPPERCORNS *Piper nigrum,*
P. cubeba and P. longum

BLACK, WHITE, GREEN, ORANGE, RED, CUBEB AND LONG

Native to the monsoon forests of the Malabar Coast, in southwest India, and Southeast Asia, black peppercorns were once valued as highly as gold and are, today, the world's most traded spice.

Peppercorns are the dried fruits (or, more precisely, drupes) of a flowering perennial vine belonging to the pepper family (*Piperaceae*). Small white flowers appear in long spikes when the plant is about five years old, and produce tightly packed drupes that are picked green and unripe, then dried on their spikes.

Black peppercorns are produced by boiling green, unripe drupes for a short time and drying them until they shrink and turn black.

Green peppercorns are unripe drupes and have a gentler, fresher, less pungent taste than black pepper. They are available fresh, dried, pickled in brine or vinegar, or freeze-dried.

Orange and red peppercorns are ripe drupes that have been preserved in the same way as green peppercorns.

White peppercorns are the seeds from inside ripe pepper drupes that have been soaked in water for a week, to soften and decompose, so that the fruit and skin are easily removed from the seed. The taste of white pepper is gentler, earthier and more musty than black pepper.

Tailed pepper (cubeb) is another species of pepper, *Piper cubeba*, easily distinguishable by the tail on the peppercorns. It is not widely available as a dried spice but is cultivated for its essential oil, which is used as a flavouring agent. Tailed pepper has an aromatic, peppery scent, and tastes like a mixture of allspice and black pepper. Once thought to be an aphrodisiac, it is used today as an antiseptic, and as an expectorant in cough remedies.

Long pepper, or pippali (*Piper longum*), is another relative in the pepper family. The fruits resemble catkins covered in tiny seeds that offer a strong, hot flavour popular in Indian, Asian and North African spice mixtures. Pippali has recently attracted medical interest because it is thought to have anti-cancer properties.

BUYING AND STORING

Peppercorns were once so valuable that suppliers often adulterated their products with cheaper alternatives, for example juniper berries, and even coal dust! Such practices are now forbidden by law, of course, but because pepper soon loses its volatile oils and aromatic qualities through evaporation and exposure to light, it is still best always to buy whole peppercorns and grind them only when required to achieve their fullest flavour. Whole peppercorns keep for a year or more, stored in an airtight container in a cool, dry place, out of direct sunlight. The peppercorns from Madagascar are considered the world's finest.

Green peppercorns in brine are best kept in the refrigerator and should be used within a month of opening. Fresh green peppercorns (when available) will keep for a few days in the refrigerator.

FOOD PROFILE

Known as the 'king of spices', black pepper is the third most frequently used cooking ingredient in the world, after water and salt. It should always be added, freshly ground, as one of the final ingredients before serving to get the most out of its flavour.

White pepper tastes great in salads and is frequently used in Chinese cuisine.

Spikes of fresh green peppercorns can be used in sauces or scattered over salads and cooked dishes, or even eaten as a piquant snack.

NUTRITIONAL PROFILE

Piperine is the chemical in pepper responsible for its spicy, hot flavour and much of its medicinal effect. It has been shown to aid absorption of nutrients, especially selenium, vitamin A and the B-group vitamins. Pepper also contains terpenes and azulene.

HEALTH PROFILE

Pepper stimulates the appetite and digestion, and speeds the transit time of food through the intestines, reducing fermentation and wind. As it causes sneezing, it can be used to relieve a cough or a congested chest, and the essential oil is used in aromatherapy to relieve pain in rheumatic conditions, as well as in the production of cosmetics. Black pepper also has a traditional reputation as a treatment for vitiligo.

NOTES:

• Pep up herbal teas by adding a few peppercorns to the brew.

Pink Peppercorns *Schinus molle* and *S. terebinthifolius*

Pink peppercorns are the dried berries of the Peruvian peppertree and the Brazilian pepper, both of which belong to the sumac family (*Anacardiaceae*). The Peruvian peppertree is native to the Andean deserts and can reach up to 15m/50ft in height. It is a fast-growing evergreen with drooping branches that bear feathery compound leaves. The Brazilian pepper is a smaller tree that has long compound leaves. Both plants bear a profusion of small white flowers that turn into dense clusters of tiny berries. These are green at first, turning red or pink as they ripen. They are then dried, roasted and called pink peppercorns. Although not botanically related to other peppercorns from the *Piper* species, they have a sweet peppery scent and flavour.

BUYING AND STORING

Pink peppercorns are easily recognizable by their bright rosy-pink colour and are usually sold dried. They will keep for several months stored in an airtight container, kept out of direct sunlight. They are also available pickled in brine, which gives them a much duller, almost greenish, tint.

FOOD PROFILE

Dried, roasted pink peppercorns have a sweet, fruity aroma when crushed and produce an interesting, sweetish, scented flavour with a hot, peppery aftertaste that is popular in Mediterranean cuisine. They are hollow with a smooth, thin skin.

Whole pink peppercorns look attractive sprinkled on top of a salad and add a sweet citrus crunch. An oil is distilled from the berries and used to add a spicy flavouring to confectionery, breads and cakes. The pink berries were used by the Incas to make a sweet, syrupy drink and the South American drink *horchatas* can be flavoured with crushed pink peppercorn berries, which are also becoming a popular addition to some craft beers and cocktails.

NUTRITIONAL PROFILE

Pink peppercorns contain volatile oil, alkyl phenols, fatty oil, flavonoids, triterpenes and gallic acid.

HEALTH PROFILE

Ripe, pink peppercorns were used by the Incas as both a spice and a medicine and have a reputation for being antibiotic, antidepressant, anti-inflammatory, astringent and antimicrobial. Traditionally, they were used to treat wounds, infections and inflammations and were taken internally as a stimulating, astringent tonic.

NOTE:
- The seeds can irritate mucous membranes in susceptible individuals if eaten in excess.

Pomegranate Seed *Punica granatum*

The pomegranate is a deciduous shrub or small tree, belonging to the loosestrife family (*Lythraceae*). Native to the Middle East region (notably Persia, or modern-day Iran), it prefers hot summers and cool winters, is drought tolerant and cultivated in many arid lands as a food crop, a spice and a medicine. It is now grown extensively in South China, India, Southeast Asia, especially Japan and Korea, southern Europe and the southern United States.

Mature pomegranate trees are distinctive and very beautiful, with multi-trunks and twisted bark, leaves that are narrow, oblong and glossy, and bright red flowers. The fruit is, in fact, a large berry, which is the size of an apple with thick red, orange or yellow inedible skin. It ripens during autumn/fall and winter, producing between 200 and 1,400 seeds, each within their own juicy aril, which in turn are arranged within a bitter white pith. The fruit may be sweet or sour, depending on its variety and ripeness, but all varieties produce an astringent juice and contain jewel-like ruby-red seeds.

The name pomegranate comes from the Latin words *pomum* (fruit) and *granatum* (seeded). In ancient Egypt, the pomegranate was an emblem of prosperity, and in ancient Persia, Greece and China it was regarded as a symbol of abundance, fertility and good luck.

BUYING AND STORING

Buy whole, fresh pomegranates with unblemished, shiny skins. The heavier the fruit, the more juice they are likely to contain, but avoid any that feel soft. Use the seeds fresh, or store in the refrigerator in an airtight container for a day or two. Pomegranate is also available dried, juiced and as a syrup. The Indian spice *anardana*, made from ground pomegranate seeds, is a souring agent in pickles and curries.

To open a fresh pomegranate, score its skin around the middle with a sharp knife. Break it open and use a teaspoon to scoop out the red seeds from the bitter white pith. This is easier to do in a bowl of water because the seeds sink and the pith floats. Freezing a pomegranate first also makes the arils easier to remove.

FOOD PROFILE

Fresh pomegranate seeds add a sweet yet astringent taste to salads, cooked dishes, breads, cakes, confectionery, smoothies, wines, liqueurs, syrups and Martini. Dried seeds are used in trail mixes, granola bars, yogurts and ice creams, and can also be covered in chocolate to make a tasty confectionery and cake decoration.

Pomegranate juice is commonly used in Middle Eastern cuisine to make marinades and sauces for a range of traditional dishes.

NUTRITIONAL PROFILE

Pomegranate seeds are rich in vitamins and minerals, especially vitamins C, K, B5, B6 and folate. They also contain tannins, alkaloids, polyphenols (including ellagic acid), pelletierine, flavonoids and anthocyanin, and are a good source of dietary fibre and antioxidants.

HEALTH PROFILE

Pomegranate is mentioned as a medicinal remedy in Egyptian papyri dating back to 1550 BC. The rind can be used as a worming remedy and the fruit may be effective in treating cystitis and other common infections such as a sore throat. The astringent quality of the juice is employed in the treatment of nosebleeds and bleeding gums, to tone up the skin and in eye drops to prevent cataracts. Pomegranate seeds are an excellent source of dietary fibre, and as such are beneficial for the digestive system and can help the body to detoxify. Because pomegranate is thought to improve the health of body cells, it may also help the immune system destroy cancer cells and thus help prevent tumours. In Ayurvedic medicine, pomegranate seeds and juice are used as a heart tonic.

NOTE:

- A glass of pomegranate juice counts as one of your vital five-a-day (although you should avoid brands with added sugar). You can also quickly increase the nutritional value of a salad or snack with a scattering of fresh pomegranate seeds.

Poppy Seed *Papaver somniferum*

The poppy seeds that we often find on our bread and breakfast rolls come from the opium poppy, although the plant's narcotic properties are not present in the ripe seeds. A member of the poppy family (*Papaveraceae*), the plant is an ornamental annual that grows up to 120cm/4ft high, with white or purple flowers and lobed, blue-tinged leaves. The poppy is native to the eastern Mediterranean and central Asia and is grown commercially mainly in China, Indo-China, India and Afghanistan, and also in Europe and North America. The tiny, hard, kidney-shaped seeds (there are more than 3,000 in a single gram) may be black, blue, brown or white, and are harvested from dried, ripe, seed capsules. They are used whole, ground into a paste or pressed as poppy seed oil.

BUYING AND STORING

Blue seeds are the most popular for use as a garnish or decoration, although black seeds are the most striking. White seeds are not so widely available but are preferred for grinding to use as a thickener.

Because of their high oil content, poppy seeds go rancid if kept for long periods at room temperature. Stored in an airtight container in the refrigerator, they will keep for up to 6 months, and up to a year when frozen. Sometimes poppy seeds are adulterated with amaranth seeds as these look similar but are less expensive.

FOOD PROFILE

Poppy seeds are a popular spice and garnish, and have a sweet, mild, nutty aroma that is released by toasting or baking. White poppy seeds are particularly popular in Indian cuisine when ground up with other spices to flavour and thicken sauces and curries. *Aloo posto* is a popular Bengali dish made with ground poppy seeds and spices cooked with potatoes, and there are many variations of these *posto* (Bengali for poppy seeds) dishes, including desserts prepared with jaggery and coconut milk.

In the West, blue and black poppy seeds are used mostly for baking and confectionery, especially for sprinkling on breads, bagels and cakes, or as a pastry filling mixed with honey, sugar and citrus zest. They are also delicious fried in a little oil and added to pasta, or sprinkled over vegetables, salads and cooked dishes just before serving. Poppy seeds are especially widely used in Jewish and eastern

European cuisines, both in baking and as a spice. Poppy seed oil has a distinct nutty flavour and makes a good addition to dressings or as a dipping oil.

NUTRITIONAL PROFILE

Poppy seeds have a high content of omega oils (particularly linoleic acid) and are thus recommended for pregnant women and nursing mothers as a healthy addition to baked foods. They are also high in calcium and contain some iron, B vitamins and dietary fibre.

HEALTH PROFILE

The opium poppy has been used since ancient times as a sedative and painkiller, and poppy seed tea is traditionally made from whole seed heads. Poppy seeds contain only a tiny amount of opium alkaloids (notably morphine and codeine), and can be used to make cough syrups. There is some evidence that poppy seeds may have anti-cancer properties and can also lower blood cholesterol levels. In Ayurvedic medicine, ground poppy seeds are used to treat skin problems.

NOTE:

- Poppy seeds can be ground with a pestle and mortar, or in a coffee mill or electric grinder. Manual poppy seed mills are also available and give a very smooth paste. The seeds are easier to grind after being toasted in a dry frying pan and mixed with a little water. For use in dough, they are best covered with boiling water and left to soak for a few hours before grinding.

Saffron 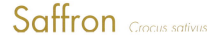 *Crocus sativus*

Saffron is the most expensive spice in the world, reputedly costing more than 10 times as much as vanilla, and 50 times more than cardamom. The spice consists of the delicate, thread-like, bright orange-red dried stigmas of the saffron crocus, which is a member of the iris family (*Iridaceae*). Also known as autumn crocus because of its late flowering, the plant grows up to 15cm/6in tall with long, thin, green leaves and blue-violet flowers. It prefers a warm and dry climate, and is grown mainly in Iran, Greece, Morocco, Spain, Turkey, Afghanistan, China, India

81

and Italy. The name 'saffron' comes from the Persian *zafaran,* meaning yellow, and, as well as being a spice, saffron has been used for centuries as a food colouring and cloth dye.

BUYING AND STORING

Available in most supermarkets and specialist food stores, saffron loses its flavour if kept too long. Always buy whole stigmas (strands) rather than ground saffron because of the risk of adulteration. Keep them stored in an airtight container, out of direct sunlight, and use within a year

The highest-quality saffron (often grown in Kashmir) has a vibrant, uniform red colour: the deeper the colour, the better the quality. Any white streaks or light patches are signs of lesser quality, and light specks in ground saffron may be a sign of adulteration. As it takes about 500 of the hand-picked and dried stigmas to make just 1g in weight, saffron is both highly labour intensive to produce and expensive to buy. This has led to it gaining the unfortunate reputation of being the most frequently adulterated spice, falsified with marigold, turmeric, paprika and other much less palatable additions.

FOOD PROFILE

Saffron is a key ingredient in Asian, Middle Eastern and Mediterranean cooking, especially to add colour and its distinctive aromatic flavour to rice dishes such as risotto and paella, and stews and casseroles such as bouillabaisse. It has long been used in northern Europe in soups, sauces, desserts, breads and cakes.

Saffron's intense colour and flavour (combined with its cost) means that only a pinch is required for a whole dish.

NUTRITIONAL PROFILE

Saffron contains volatile oils including safranal, cineole, phenathenol, pinene, borneol, geraniol, limonene and linalool. It is also rich in carotenoids such as alpha-crocin, zeaxanthin, lycopene and beta-carotene, and also vitamin B2 (riboflavin), calcium, magnesium, manganese, potassium, iron, selenium and zinc.

HEALTH PROFILE

Saffron is valued as a medicinal herb for its antioxidant, immune-boosting, antiseptic, anti-convulsant, expectorant, digestive, antidepressant, sedative and mildly narcotic properties. It is used to treat coughs and bronchitis, and also as a remedy for insomnia, stress and depression. It should not be taken medicinally during pregnancy.

NOTE:
- To achieve an even colouring, soak saffron strands in hot water for a few minutes and then add both the saffron and the liquid to the dish and stir in well.

Salt *Sodium chloride*

Although not a spice by traditional definition, salt is probably the best known and most widely used seasoning in the kitchen. It is produced either by evaporating seawater, or by extraction from salt mines that provide access to the mineral content of ancient evaporated salt lakes. There is evidence that salt mines existed as far back as Neolithic times, at least 8,000 years ago.

Unrefined sea salt has a light grey colour and is considered to have a richer flavour than rock salt due to it also containing magnesium, calcium, sulphates and traces of algae. White sea salt has been refined to remove some of these substances.

Rock salt, or halite, is commonly used as table salt, having been refined to remove impurities. It usually contains anti-caking agents to prevent clumping and, sometimes, iodine to help prevent thyroid problems such as goitre. Fluoride may also be added to table salt to help prevent tooth decay. Sea salt and kosher salt contain no additives.

As well as being the world's most ubiquitous flavouring, salt is also significant as a food preservative, especially historically in the days before refrigeration. We know from ancient records that people used salt to dehydrate foodstuffs and so prevent the growth of harmful bacteria. Salted foods have long been a part of people's diets all over the world and still are today. Even the Egyptians used salt as part of the mummification process.

Such was the value of salt that wars were fought over it and ownership of it could determine power. Though cheap and widely available today, salt was once valued more highly than gold for its rarity; in fact that the word 'salary' derives from the Latin *salis*, meaning salt. However, salt has become a standard ingredient in many processed foods and we are increasingly aware that too much salt in the diet can raise blood pressure and increase the risk of strokes and heart attacks. Salt is also significant in many industrial and manufacturing processes.

BUYING AND STORING

Refined table salt and fine and coarse sea salt are readily available in most grocery stores and supermarkets. Other varieties are kosher salt, which has large irregular flakes; fleur de sel, the top layer of sea salt deposits; and black salt, which contains lava and tastes of sulphur. Store salt in a dry, airtight container (but not silverware as sodium chloride reacts with silver, turning it green). It lasts indefinitely.

FOOD PROFILE

Salt enhances the flavours of the food we eat. The word 'salad' comes from the old habit of salting raw greens to give them more taste. It has no smell but provides a strong, almost acidic taste and should be added to dishes only in small amounts to avoid overpowering the flavours of other ingredients.

NUTRITIONAL PROFILE

Salt is important to all living things and a certain amount is necessary for human survival. It helps to regulate our internal fluid balance and plays a role in muscle contraction and relaxation and the transmission of nerve impulses.

HEALTH PROFILE

The amount of salt in the body is regulated by the kidneys. If the kidneys cannot get rid of excess salt (because of kidney disease or too much salt in the diet), it starts to build up in the bloodstream, which can lead to high blood pressure, oedema and even heart failure and stroke. While everyone has a different level of tolerance to salt, most authorities recommend limiting total dietary salt intake to no more than 2.3g/ less than ½ teaspoon, per day (and less as you get older or if you are suffering from kidney or heart disease). In this respect, it is important to count the hidden salt found in all processed, fast and prepared foods, breads, snacks, meat and egg dishes, breakfast cereals, pizza, cold meats, bacon, shellfish, cheese, other dairy products and many condiments.

Externally, salt is a cleanser and detoxifier. Salt water can be used in baths, mouthwashes and gargles to deal with local infections.

- Put a few grains of uncooked rice in a salt shaker to avoid caking. Alternatives to salt include soy sauce, onion powder, lemon juice, garlic powder and seaweed.

Sansho *Zanthoxylum piperitum*

Sansho, also known as Japanese pepper, is one of the few spices commonly used in Japanese cookery. It is not a true pepper but a berry produced by a Japanese variety of prickly ash; a spiny, aromatic, deciduous shrub or small tree belonging to the citrus family (*Rutaceae*). The sansho bush prefers a fertile soil and a sunny but shady position, and is grown commercially in Japan, South Korea and China.

Sansho flowers grow in clusters and form bright, lime-green berries that turn red as they ripen in the autumn/fall. Young leaves and shoots herald the coming of spring and are used as a garnish, or to make a sauce for seafood dishes. The mature berries, sometimes misleadingly referred to as sansho peppercorns, are an important flavouring in Japanese cuisine, where they are one of the seven key ingredients in shichimi togarashi, a popular Japanese spice mixture (see next page). Sansho is also sometimes used as one of the ingredients in Chinese five-spice mixtures.

Despite its name, sansho pepper is not actually a pepper, nor is it peppery in flavour, and it should not be confused with black or pink peppercorns. The spice is closely related to Szechuan pepper (see pages 88–90).

BUYING AND STORING

Sansho is mostly available in ground powder form, or occasionally as whole berries from Oriental grocery stores and specialist food retailers.

FOOD PROFILE

Having an earthy, tangy, lemony and light, spicy flavour, sansho is used traditionally to flavour miso soup, noodles, rice, pickles, rice crackers and teriyaki. It is especially popular sprinkled over rich fatty dishes. Ground sansho is an essential flavouring in the popular spice mixture *shichimi togarashi*, combined with ground dried chilli, nori, dried tangerine peel, white and black sesame seeds and poppy seeds, which is served as a table condiment for sprinkling over dishes.

Often the ground ripe berries are simply mixed together with salt and used as a seasoning; unripe green sansho berries can also be pickled and eaten with soy sauce. Sansho leaves are highly aromatic when bruised and can be eaten raw in salads or added as a garnish.

NUTRITIONAL PROFILE
Sansho berries contain volatile oils including geraniol, dipentene and citral, as well as sanshool (responsible for their pungency), and various flavonoids, including quercetin and hesperidin.

HEALTH PROFILE
Sansho is considered a warming, stimulating spice. In Chinese medicine it is thought to benefit the spleen and stomach, to stimulate digestion and relieve cold digestive complaints. It has antibacterial and antifungal properties, and can be used as a worming remedy against intestinal parasites. It also has a diuretic and blood-pressure-lowering effect, and can be used as a local anaesthetic.

NOTES:
- Sansho is used as a flavouring in the ceremonial wine known as *toso*, which is traditionally drunk in Japan to celebrate New Year.
- *Tsukudani*, a popular condiment, is made by simmering kombu or wakame seaweed with sansho, soy sauce and rice wine. It is good served chilled to flavour steamed rice, but should be used sparingly as its flavour is very intense.

STAR ANISE *Illicium verum*

Star anise are the dried fruits of an aromatic, medium-tall, evergreen tree belonging to the schisandra family (*Schisandraceae*, formerly part of the magnolia family). The tree starts to bear fruit when it is about six years old, and carries on producing for up to a hundred years. The fruits consist of eight hard elliptical seedpods, called points, arranged in a star shape, which are picked before they ripen. Dried in the sun, they harden and become aromatic as they turn dark brown. Each seedpod is hollow and houses a single, shiny brown seed.

The plant is native to southwest China and northeast Vietnam, and although there is some commercial production in Vietnam, Indo-China, Japan and Australia, 90% of world supply comes from China.

Star anise has a long history of use in Chinese medicine and Asian cookery, and was introduced to Europe in the 17th century, where it became popular as a flavouring agent in preserves, syrups, cordials, pastilles and cough mixtures.

Star anise is not related to aniseed or fennel (see pages 21–22 and 45–47) although it has a similar taste and fragrance.

BUYING AND STORING

Buy pre-packed, whole, unbroken star anise from Asian food stores, health food stores, spice merchants or supermarkets to be sure it has not been contaminated with Japanese star anise (see Warning on page 88). Store the spice in an airtight jar in a cool, dark place, and discard when the flavour begins to fade (usually after about a year). Once ground, the flavour of star anise diminishes within a few months, so it is best only to buy small quantities of pre-ground star anise if you cannot find the whole spice.

FOOD PROFILE

Star anise has a sweetly pungent, slightly bitter, liquorice flavour, which is stronger than aniseed and so should be used sparingly. It can be added whole to soups, casseroles and stews, or ground to a powder for use in stir-fries, and to flavour cakes and breads. An essential spice in Chinese cuisine, star anise is a key ingredient in Chinese five-spice powder (see page 117), and is also a popular feature in Vietnamese dishes such as the noodle soup, *Pho Bo*. It is also an important ingredient in Malay, Indonesian and Indian curries and spice mixtures, including garam masala, biryani and chai, and in the West it is used in baking, confectionery, fruit compotes, preserves, liqueurs and alcoholic beverages such as pastis, anisette and absinthe.

NUTRITIONAL PROFILE

Star anise contains anethole, shikimic acid, flavonoids, sesquiterpenes, lignans and caryophyllene.

HEALTH PROFILE

The shikimic acid contained in star anise seeds is a strong antiviral agent and a primary ingredient in the synthesis of antiviral drugs such as Tamiflu. Recent bird flu and swine flu epidemics caused the price of star anise to soar as drug companies bought up vast quantities in order to meet the surge in worldwide demand for antiviral drugs.

Star anise is a warming, stimulating herb used in traditional Chinese medicine to relieve cold stagnation, to balance the flow of *Qi* and to relieve pain. It is a traditional remedy for arthritis and digestive complaints, and has potent antimicrobial properties due, in part, to the presence of anethole, which is effective against bacteria, fungus and some yeasts. Its immune-stimulating, antimicrobial and antioxidant properties, together with a gentle painkilling and sedative effect, make star anise a perfect remedy to give young children to relieve colic, and also to treat respiratory problems such as bronchitis, cough and asthma. It is also a useful insect repellent.

NOTES:

- Try sprinkling ground star anise on root vegetables before baking, or add a whole star anise to sweet potato, pumpkin or leek dishes to enhance their flavour. Star anise also brings out the sweetness of cooked and raw tomatoes.
- A cup of herb tea looks and tastes even better with a star anise added.

WARNING:

- It is important not to confuse Chinese star anise (*Illicium verum*) with Japanese star anise (*Illicium anisatum*), which is toxic. Japanese star anise has more pointed, more irregular fruits and is strictly not for internal use.

Szechuan Pepper *Zanthoxylum bungeanum*

Szechuan pepper comes from a number of *Zanthoxylum* species in the citrus family (*Rutaceae*) and is closely related to sansho (Japanese pepper, see pages 85–86). It is also known in Chinese as mountain pepper, wild peppercorn, flower pepper and Chinese prickly ash. A small deciduous shrub, native to eastern

China and Taiwan, Szechuan pepper grows up to 4m/13ft tall and has large knobs on its trunk and branches, and short spines on its stems and leaves. It prefers moist soil but grows equally well in sun and shade. The flowers appear in spring in yellowish-green clusters that turn into tiny reddish-brown berries in the autumn/fall. The ripe berries release a small black seed and it is the remaining seedpod husk that is collected for use as a spice and medicine. These so-called peppercorns resemble tiny rust-coloured beech nuts with thin stems.

BUYING AND STORING

Szechuan pepper is available as whole berries or ground, and should be stored in an airtight container in a cool place out of direct sunlight.

FOOD PROFILE

Regarded as one of the oldest established spices in Chinese cuisine, Szechuan pepper is often used in combination with star anise and ginger, and it is becoming increasingly well known in Western cooking for its unique, spicy aroma. It is one of the key ingredients in Chinese five-spice powder (see page 117) and has an aromatic, gently pungent, slightly lemony, spicy, anise-like taste and produces a fizzy, tingly, numbing effect on the tongue. It can be mixed with salt as a traditional Chinese condiment, or soaked in oil and used in stir-fries, noodles and rice dishes, together with ginger, jaggery and vinegar.

NUTRITIONAL PROFILE

Szechuan pepper contains volatile oils, including geraniol, linalool, limonene-cineol, as well as flavonoids and terpene alkaloids or alkamides, including sanshool.

HEALTH PROFILE

Szechuan pepper has a warming, stimulating, local anaesthetic quality and is used traditionally to cool fevers, and as a vasodilator to lower blood pressure. It can also relieve stomach ache and indigestion, and has a reputation as a worming remedy against tapeworm.

NOTES:

- Toasting Szechuan peppercorns brings out their flavour and makes the seedpods easier to crush.

- For a traditional Szechuan taste, add toasted seedpods mixed with chilli at the last minute to Chinese sauces and hotpots.

Tamarind *Tamarindus indica*

The spice tamarind is the fruit pulp of the Indian date, a tropical tree belonging to the legume family (*Leguminosae*). The tamarind tree grows incredibly tall and can live for 200 years or more. It is graceful and slow-growing with a broad, ash-grey trunk and pinnate leaves with up to 40 oval leaflets. The flowers are yellow, arranged in clusters, and the fruits are long, bean-like, reddish-brown pods that contain 6–12 seeds enclosed in a sticky pulp.

As well as growing wild throughout India and much of South Asia, the tree is cultivated in tropical Africa, northern Australia, Mexico, Taiwan and China, and has also become naturalized in the Middle East. Tamarind is valued as a souring agent in Indian, Thai and Jamaican cuisine and has a similar effect on foods as lemons and limes. The main commercial producers and consumers today are Mexico and India.

BUYING AND STORING

Tamarind is widely available in major supermarkets and in Asian food stores either in hard, pressed fibrous slabs or as a paste. The dried pods are also available in some Asian stores and markets and fresh pods may be available when in season. Both the slabs and the paste will keep for up to a year and the dried pods will keep for much longer, but the slabs and dried pods need to be soaked before use. Tamarind paste can be used straight from the jar, and the pulp from fresh pods can be separated from the seeds and eaten raw.

FOOD PROFILE

The pulp from tamarind is dark red-brown, stringy, moist and sugary with a slightly fruity, lemony aroma, and a refreshing sweet, yet very sour taste. It adds character to curries and to sauces, pickles and chutneys, and is also excellent for preserves because of its high pectin content. Tamarind syrup can be used to make a refreshing lemonade and is an important ingredient in Worcestershire sauce.

NUTRITIONAL PROFILE

Tamarind contains geraniol, limonene and methyl salicylate, as well as sugars, pectin, fibre, omega-6 fatty acid, vitamins B1, B2, B3 and C, iron, magnesium, phosphorus, potassium and plant acids such as malic and tartaric acid.

HEALTH PROFILE

Tamarind has a cooling effect and can be used to treat fevers, as well as simply for cooling down on a hot day. It is a traditional remedy for respiratory disorders and constipation, and can be taken as a gargle to ease a sore throat. Externally, it can be applied as an antiseptic.

NOTES:

- Soak tamarind slabs in hot water for 10 minutes, then mash and pass through a sieve/fine-mesh strainer before use.
- Tamarind juice with finely chopped garlic and ginger, and the juice of half an orange makes a wonderful barbecue basting sauce.
- Tamarind makes an excellent natural polish for copper and brass. Sprinkle a chunk of tamarind with salt, moisten and rub directly onto the object. Rinse and dry with a cloth.

TURMERIC *Curcuma longa*

Turmeric is the rhizome, or underground rootstalk, of a perennial, tropical plant belonging to the ginger (*Zingiberaceae*) family. As such, it looks like ginger and is prepared and used in a similar way: peeled, then sliced, grated, chopped or ground to a paste. Alternatively, the roots can be boiled for several hours, then dried and ground to a powder to produce the familiar vibrant golden-yellow spice that is readily available today in most supermarkets.

The name 'turmeric' may come from the Latin *terra merita* meaning 'merit of the earth'. As well as being valued for its aroma, flavour and vibrant colour, turmeric has also long been prized in Indian and Ayurvedic medicine as an important medicine and disinfectant. It is believed to have the quality of fire, or *pitta*, giving it a stimulating, cleansing effect. It is also held to be auspicious and holy, and plays a significant role in many Hindu and Buddhist religious ceremonies, symbolizing power and purification. Traditionally, the golden-yellow textile dye that is made from turmeric is used to colour the robes of Buddhist monks.

Native to tropical Asia, turmeric is now grown in India, Sri Lanka, China, Taiwan, Indonesia, Peru, the West Indies, Africa and Australia. In medieval times, when turmeric was first brought to Europe, it was known as Indian saffron and often substituted as a cheaper alternative to genuine *Crocus sativus*. But while saffron and turmeric do tint foods a similar golden colour, their taste, aroma and medicinal qualities are distinctly different.

BUYING AND STORING

Fresh turmeric can be found in specialist Asian food stores and gourmet groceries, but it is much more widely available as a dried ground, golden-yellow spice powder. It is best bought in small quantities and stored in an airtight container in a dry place, out of direct sunlight.

FOOD PROFILE

Turmeric is used to give an attractive vibrant yellow colour to curries, sauces and condiments, and imparts a distinct, earthy, dry and slightly peppery bitter flavour. It is a key ingredient in many South Asian and Middle Eastern savoury dishes and plays a featuring role in most curry powder mixtures. Considered to be an excellent aid to digestion, turmeric is frequently added to lentil and bean dishes in Indian cookery. In areas where turmeric grows, the fresh leaves of the plant are sometimes used to wrap around food before cooking to add extra flavour. They are also available pickled.

In the West, turmeric is mostly valued as a dry spice for its characteristic rich, bright yellow colouring and mellow flavour. It is added to drinks, ice creams, cheeses, butter, margarine, yogurts, confectionery, icings, breads, cakes, mustards, stocks and sauces, often in the guise of E100, the code applied to turmeric when it is used as a food colouring agent. Turmeric is also used in cosmetics and as a clothing and general purpose dye.

NUTRITIONAL PROFILE

Turmeric contains high levels of curcumin, as well as sterols, resins and volatile oils. It is rich in vitamins C, B3 and B6, and also magnesium, manganese, potassium, copper, iron, zinc and omega-6 fatty acids.

HEALTH PROFILE

Turmeric has been valued in Chinese and Ayurvedic medicine for centuries as a remedy for stomach and liver problems, for inflammation and to treat wounds and tumours. It is known to be a good antiseptic, effective against a variety of fungal and bacterial infections, and research has confirmed that it may also help to inhibit the spread of cancer by destroying mutant cells and can enhance the effects of chemotherapy and radiation therapy.

Consequently, turmeric has become the focus of much medical interest and research in recent years. It is thought to have significant potential in the fight against degenerative diseases such as Alzheimer's, type-2 diabetes, arthritis and pancreatic disorders. The active ingredient attracting most attention is curcumin, which is a strong antioxidant capable of protecting cells against free radical damage. Curcumin also reduces histamine levels, and may increase the production of cortisone in the body. A double-blind trial found that turmeric was more effective than both placebo and non-steroidal anti-inflammatory drugs (NSAIDs) in the relief of inflammation after surgery, perhaps opening the way to the development of a range of new anti-inflammatory medications that could have significantly fewer side effects.

Turmeric is also used as an anti-ageing remedy to soften the skin and to ease the symptoms of psoriasis. Freshly grated turmeric root can also be applied externally in various hair conditioners, purifying skin wraps and face masks.

NOTE:
- Try making your own simple health boosters and remedies:

Turmeric Natural Health Supplement

1 tsp ground turmeric   1–2 tsp olive oil
a pinch of freshly ground black pepper

Mix the turmeric and black pepper with enough olive oil to make a paste. Eat spread on a slice of bread or with yogurt.

Pain-relieving Turmeric Paste

1 tsp ground turmeric   1 tsp almond oil, plus extra for wiping

Mix the turmeric and oil to a smooth paste. Apply to the head, neck and shoulders to relieve headache, or to the back or legs to relieve arthritic pain. Leave in place for 5 minutes, then wipe off with almond oil.

WARNING:

- Remember that turmeric is a strong yellow dye that stains.

VANILLA *Vanilla planifolia*

Vanilla is the only edible orchid fruit, and although there are around 150 types of vanilla orchid, only a few are grown successfully commercially: flat-leaved vanilla, Tahitian vanilla, West Indian vanilla and Bourbon vanilla. Flat-leaved vanilla is native to Mexico, which was once the world's sole supplier; Tahitian vanilla is from French Polynesia; West Indian vanilla is produced in the Caribbean and Central/South America; and Bourbon vanilla is produced in India and the Indian Ocean Islands.

The vanilla orchid is a vine of the orchid family (*Orchidaceae*) that thrives at high altitude and prefers a hot tropical climate. Cultivated for centuries by the Aztecs of Mexico, vanilla was introduced into Europe, along with chocolate, by the Spanish conquistador Hernán Cortés in the early 16th century.

The plant is self-fertile, but cultivating vanilla is labour intestive as the flowers last only one day and must be pollinated in order to bear fruit. A successful method of hand-pollination, which is still used today, was discovered by a 12-year-old slave boy called Edmond Albius in 1841 on the French Île de la Réunion. Mastery of this delicate technque made it possible for vanilla cultivation and production to be succesful in locations other than Mexico, which had held a monopoly on vanilla production until the 1840s. The tropical orchids were transplanted successfully to Mauritius, Polynesia and Madagascar, and now the main vanilla producers are Indonesia and Madagascar. Vanilla production, however, is still an extremely labour-intensive business.

Mature plants flower and bear fruit after about four years, and the long, thin fruit pods, which contain thousands of tiny black seeds, take about five months to ripen. Harvested pods/beans are cured in a process of fermentation and drying designed to preserve their volatile oil content, and the resulting cured pods/beans are tough, slender and dark brown in colour. Vanilla may have a frosting of crystals called 'givre', containing vanillin, the main active aromatic ingredient; woody vanilla lacks givre and is shorter, lighter in colour, drier, more brittle and stronger-tasting.

After saffron and cardamom, vanilla is the world's third most expensive spice, but is also one of the most widely used flavourings. As a consequence, artificial vanillin was developed in the 1870s, and it is this synthetic substitute that is most commonly used commercially in the food and perfume industries.

BUYING AND STORING

For the finest vanilla flavour, look out for vanilla from Madagascar and Mexico, and expect to pay a high price. Real vanilla costs about 200 times that of its artificial substitute. Fortunately, whole vanilla pods/beans can be reused several times over, and will last at least 6 months with this method of storage: steep the pod/bean in hot water, then leave it to cool for an hour. Remove the pod/bean and use the liquid to poach fruit or make a syrup. Rinse and dry the pod/bean and store it in a dry, airtight container, kept in the dark. Alternatively, bury it in a jar of sugar and gain the added bonus of having a ready supply of mellow, fragrant vanilla-flavoured sugar. For the most intense vanilla flavouring, split the pod/bean with a sharp knife and scrape out some of the seeds

Ground vanilla, or vanilla powder, is available commercially and imparts a stronger flavour than infusing a whole pod/bean. It should be used very sparingly and mixed with a little water before adding to recipes.

Vanilla extract is made by soaking chopped pods/beans in alcohol (minimum 35%), and the stronger the alcohol, the better the quality of the extract. This is the best alternative to vanilla pods/beans.

FOOD PROFILE

Vanilla has a pure, sweet and distinctly powerful aromatic flavour and a complex, flowery scent. The mellow, sweet taste and evocative fragrance of vanilla is unrivalled as a favourite ice cream flavouring, and it is commonly used to enhance the taste and appeal of many sweet foods and drinks, liqueurs, desserts, confectionery and chocolate. Indeed, vanilla is probably the strongest contender for the title of 'world's favourite flavour'.

The term 'French vanilla' refers to the French method of making creamy caramel desserts and ice creams from a vanilla-flavoured custard. It sometimes refers to a particularly buttery vanilla aroma.

Synthetically produced vanillin is much cheaper than the real thing and far more commonplace, now meeting the majority of the world's demand. Artificial vanillin has a more heavy fragrance and a somewhat bitter aftertaste.

NUTRITIONAL PROFILE
The active ingredients in vanilla include vanillin, vanillic acid and benzoic acid, small amounts of B-complex vitamins such as niacin and riboflavin, and trace minerals.

HEALTH PROFILE
Interesting new research from around the world suggests that vanillin may inhibit the growth of cancer cells and limit the formation of metastasis by inhibiting their blood supply. It has also been shown to reduce DNA mutations and to influence the genes that control the growth and lifespan of cancer cells.

Vanilla is widely used in the production of perfumes and cosmetics, and has a traditional, though unproven, reputation as an aphrodisiac.

NOTE:
- Synthetic vanilla is produced from guaiacol, a wood derivative, and is much less expensive and more easily obtainable than the real thing. Unsurprisingly, synthetic vanilla flavouring is used in at least 75% of processed foods and products described as being vanilla. It is also a popular ingredient in perfumes, cosmetics, medicines, animal foods and cleaning products.

WARNING:
- Vanillin can trigger migraine and should be avoided by sufferers.

Wasabi *Wasabia japonica*

Also known as Japanese horseradish, wasabi is a member of the cabbage family (*Brassicaceae*), and comes from a perennial plant, that produces rounded leaves and a long, pale green, horseradish-like root. Wasabi is described as Japanese horseradish because it has similarities in shape and taste to Western horseradish, but it is only distantly related and wasabi has a much hotter, richer, more mustardy flavour.

A traditional spice and a highly prized condiment in Japanese cuisine, wasabi can be hard to grow, needing just the right amount of light and fresh, flowing water to thrive. Its natural habitat is along the marshy banks of cool, shaded mountain streams, so cultivation on a commercial scale is difficult and has resulted in wasabi becoming expensive and increasingly scarce. As a result, most wasabi eaten in Japan today is imported from China, Taiwan and New Zealand, and the wasabi sold in the West is frequently an imitation made from horseradish, mustard, cornflour/cornstarch and chlorophyll, or an artificial green colouring. True wasabi is never cheap to buy.

BUYING AND STORING

Fresh wasabi is very difficult to find, but it is widely available dried and ground into a fine green powder, which is mixed with a little water to form wasabi paste. The dried powder keeps its flavour better than pre-mixed pastes, so it is best to buy the powder and make up the paste only when required. Leave the paste to stand for a few minutes after rehydrating to let the full flavour develop. Once exposed to the air, the heat and flavour of wasabi deteriorates quite rapidly.

If you do manage to find fresh wasabi root, the brownish-green skin should be removed and the pale green flesh should be ground as finely as possible. It should be used within 15–20 minutes, before the fierce flavour evaporates. If well wrapped and kept in the refrigerator, wasabi powder will keep for up to 2 years.

FOOD PROFILE

Wasabi paste is the perfect flavour enhancer for sushi, and makes a delicious addition to dressings, marinades, dips and sauces. Most sashimi (raw fish) dishes come adorned with a tiny amount of wasabi paste or grated wasabi, which is mixed with soy sauce for dipping.

NUTRITIONAL PROFILE

Wasabi is very high in vitamin C, and also contains vitamins B1, B2 and B6 together with calcium, magnesium, phosphorus, potassium, zinc, manganese, fibre, glucosinolates, isothiocyanates (including methyl-ITC) and carotenoids.

HEALTH PROFILE

Wasabi is a potent natural antibacterial and antifungal remedy, and research has shown that it may be able to not only kill microorganisms (including *staphylococcus* and *E. coli*), but also inhibit cancer cell growth by stimulating the immune system.

As anyone that has eaten wasabi paste will know, the taste goes powerfully up the nose, which makes wasabi an effective remedy for sinusitis, asthma, bronchitis and other conditions where mucus needs to be dissolved. Wasabi is also thought to be an excellent detox aid, stimulating the liver and digestion and possibly helping to reduce blood fat levels

Zedoary *Curcuma zedoaria*

Also known as white turmeric, *gajutsu* and *kentjur*, zedoary spice is made from the large root of a perennial aromatic tropical plant which produces yellow flowers and long fragrant leaves. Zedoary is a member of the ginger family (*Zingiberaceae*), and a close relative of turmeric, galangal and ginger. Similarly, the source of this spice is the fleshy yellow rhizome, which is sliced and dried before use.

Zedoary is widely cultivated in the subtropical wet forests of the Indian subcontinent, Thailand, Japan, China and Brazil, but it is rarely exported. Although it was highly valued and used as a medicinal and aromatic spice in Europe in the Middle Ages, its popularity in the West was overtaken by ginger.

BUYING AND STORING

Dried zedoary is available in specialist Chinese food stores and Asian supermarkets, either as a powder or in hard, dried, thin slices. It should be stored in an airtight container out of direct sunlight and used within a year.

Fresh zedoary root is available from Asian food stores, and it is also possible to buy it from online spice suppliers. If you have difficulty buying it fresh, you can substitute 1 tablespoon of fresh zedoary root with 1 teaspoon of dried.

FOOD PROFILE

Zedoary smells of mango and tastes like ginger but with a pronounced bitter aftertaste. It can be used fresh in salads and stews, or ground and added to curry pastes and pickles.

NUTRITIONAL PROFILE

Zedoary contains volatile oils, including camphor, as well as curcumin, sesquiterpenes, starch gums and phytosterols.

HEALTH PROFILE

A traditional Ayurvedic remedy for menstrual pain, discharge, intestinal worms, indigestion, colds, coughs and fever, zedoary also has a modern application as an antiseptic, anti-inflammatory, antifungal and antibacterial against gram-positive bacteria (such as *staphylococcus*), gram-negative bacteria (such as *salmonella* and *E. coli*), and yeasts (such as *candida*). Also, it can be applied externally to promote wound healing, and zedoary oil is also used in bitter tonics, soaps and perfumes.

NOTES:

- To make a digestive tisane, add 1 tablespoon of sliced zedoary root to 250ml/8fl oz/1 cup of boiling water. Leave it to infuse for 20 minutes, then drain and drink 30 minutes before meals (one or two cups per day).
- Zedoary is rich in starch and can be used as a substitute for arrowroot in baking.

COOKING WITH SPICES

Cooking with spices is akin to using magic! These extraordinary
ingredients, each in their own way, have the ability not only
to enhance and enrich the flavour, appearance and fragrance,
but also to make foods healthier, easier to digest and longer-lasting.
So one of the easiest ways to follow Hippocrates' recommendation
to make your food your medicine and your medicine your food,
is to keep the contents of your spice cupboard well stocked and
well used. The recipes that follow are developed to suit all dietary
preferences. I myself advocate and follow a plant-based diet,
rich in organic produce.

INTRODUCTION

In ancient times there were no Recommended Daily Allowances (RDA, see page 233) to instruct people on what and what not to eat, nor were there any refrigerators or freezers, or sell-by and use-by dates. Yet, by judiciously using their tastebuds and passing on recipes and nutritional wisdom from generation to generation, our ancestors survived and thrived, and made it possible for us to live on Earth today.

In ancient societies, nutrition and medicine were thought of as one science, just as astrology and astronomy were considered two faces of the same truth. In the continuing Indian tradition of Ayurveda, for example, there are six different tastes that should be eaten at each meal, not only to satisfy hunger but also to give a feeling of fullness, to ease digestion and to soothe body, mind and spirit. These tastes are sweet (for example, jaggery or vanilla); sour (tamarind or kaffir lime leaves); salty; pungent (pepper or garlic); bitter (fenugreek or cumin); and astringent (pomegranate or turmeric). These days, many synthetic flavourings and flavour enhancers are added to processed food to make them more palatable. Spices do the same job, but instead of being a potential health hazard, they can bring out the best in natural foods and transform simple dishes into epicurean delights.

Spiced food does not necessarily mean fiery hot food; there are spices to suit all palates, and all are beneficial to health. Children tend to have more sensitive taste buds and often are not keen on highly spiced dishes. However, they can enjoy the wonderful flavours of spices when applied in modest amounts simply to enhance, rather than dominate, the tastes of other ingredients. When people with different taste preferences are eating together, it is a good idea to make up a selection of spice mixtures, preserves, chutneys or condiments beforehand, and serve them alongside the main dishes. Such a choice allows individual diners to add as much or as little extra spice as they prefer, in just the same way as they would add salt or pepper.

Spices can add a new dimension to hot and cold drinks. Making a spiced tea to give warmth and help prevent a cold is cheaper and much more satisfying than reaching for an over-the-counter medicine. Adding aromatic spices to desserts, cakes and confectionery can also reduce the quantity of sugar required to sweeten a dish.

I hope that these recipes will inspire you to expand your selection of spices and start exploring their many attributes. I have found that the more I venture into new and different taste experiences, the more interesting my day-to-day cooking has become. As I have become a more experienced spice-chef, I have also learnt that creating contrasts in flavour produces more nourishing and more satisfying meals, which are both more wholesome and more enjoyable to eat.

On a practical note, I recommend that you use whole spices, store them out of direct sunlight in airtight containers, and grind them only when required. Their active ingredients are released by the processes of crushing, grinding and heating, and soon start to fade.

Diet can be a contentious issue, and it is important to respect other people's food choices. My way of promoting peace around the dining table is to ensure that my recipes are easy to adapt to many different diet styles so that everyone can enjoy eating together. My mother was a strong believer in self-sufficiency – so I have clear memories of half-pigs being delivered and prepared for later use, while produce from the forest, fields and garden also filled the freezer and the larder shelves. When I turned vegan, my family was at a loss to work out how to include me in their meals. This gave me the idea of writing recipes that include alternative ingredient suggestions for different diet styles. It has worked well for us, and I hope you will have fun doing the same, especially if you have a vegan in the family!

The weight of evidence is that lower meat consumption is associated with better health. If you do eat meat, choose organic as the higher up the food chain you are, the more vulnerable you become to the effects of chemical adulteration. Tofu, quorn, tempeh and seitan, together with pulses, nuts and vegetables, make cheaper, and often healthier, alternatives to meat. Most of these products are available, fresh, frozen and dried and I suggest them as alternatives in many recipes.

Cow's milk contains plenty of vitamins and minerals, but also contains proteins, hormones, sugars and fats that are not so easily digested by humans. In some people, cow's milk may cause digestive disorders and provoke immune reactions. I recommend soy, almond, coconut, hazelnut, oat, rice and hemp milk products as good alternatives, and leave you to decide.

Olive oil is an excellent all-round choice for general cooking and dressings. Coconut oil, used sparingly, is good for baking and frying, as is rapeseed oil. Nut and seed oils are best reserved for dressings.

NOTE:

- The nutritional and calorie information for each recipe applies only to the ingredients listed (based on the first ingredient listed if alternatives are given), and not to any alternative options or additional serving suggestions (in *italic*).

SPICE BLENDS

Hot Peppercorn Mix

A combination of whole peppercorns looks fantastic displayed in a clear pepper mill, and is a quick way to add heat, piquancy and zest to any dish. For more colour and fruitiness, and less heat, replace the melegueta and sansho pepper with pink and green peppercorns, and the Szechuan peppercorns with allspice.

Preparation time: 5 minutes

To fill a 70ml/2¼fl oz jar

1 tbsp black peppercorns

1 tbsp white peppercorns

1 tbsp Szechuan peppercorns

1 tbsp melegueta pepper

1 tbsp sansho berries

Mix the peppercorns together and store in an airtight container or a pepper mill. Grind as required over dishes as a condiment, or add to soups, casseroles, marinades, stir-fries and bakes.

NUTRIENT BALANCE (per portion)
17% protein, 9% fat, 56% carbohydrate, 18% fibre

VITAMINS AND MINERALS (percentage of RDA)
Potassium 1%, calcium 1%, magnesium 1%, iron 2%, copper 2%, manganese 6%

HEALTH BENEFITS
Strongly antioxidant | stimulates digestion | helps increase metabolism | potential anti-diabetic action | stimulates circulation

Jamaican Jerk Marinade

Jerk marinade has two main ingredients: chilli and allspice. Scotch bonnets are authentic, but jalapeños can be substituted. Use the mixture to marinade meat, fish, tofu or root vegetables for at least 2 hours before cooking. If time is tight, you can use orange marmalade in place of the caramelized oranges. The jerk is best made in advance and will keep for several days stored in an airtight container in the refrigerator.

Preparation and cooking time: 20 minutes, plus cooling

Makes 400ml/14fl oz/1⅔ cups

3 tbsp muscovado/soft brown sugar

1 tbsp coconut oil

1 orange, unpeeled, sliced

5cm/2in piece of root ginger, finely chopped

5 fresh chillies, deseeded and chopped

4 spring onions/scallions, chopped

1 tbsp honey

1 tsp dried thyme

1 tsp French mustard

2 tbsp ground allspice

3 tbsp vinegar

1 tsp sea salt

Dissolve the sugar in 2 tablespoons boiling water and pour into a heated frying pan. Reduce the liquid on a medium heat, tilting the pan, until the water has evaporated and the sugar starts to caramelize. Add the coconut oil and heat through, then add the orange slices and spread evenly in the caramel. Turn after 2 minutes so both sides are soaked in caramel. Remove from the heat and leave to cool. Transfer to a food processor or blender, add the remaining ingredients and blend until smooth. Leave to stand for at least 4 hours to let the flavours develop.

NUTRIENT BALANCE (per portion)
5% protein, 25% fat, 63% carbohydrate, 7% fibre

VITAMINS AND MINERALS (percentage of RDA)
Vitamin A 2%, C 18%, B1 2%, B3 2%, B6 2%, folate 5%, potassium 5%, calcium 5%, magnesium 3%, iron 8%, zinc 2%, copper 4%, manganese 6%

HEALTH BENEFITS
Antioxidant | antibiotic | immunity booster | stimulates digestion and circulation

Berbere

A fiery blend from Ethiopia, berbere is made as a dry spice mix, or as a paste
with the addition of fresh garlic, ginger, oil and wine.

Preparation and cooking time: 15 minutes, plus cooling

To fill a 100ml/3½fl oz jar

1 tsp galangal slices	2 whole cloves
1 tsp nigella seeds	1 cinnamon stick, broken up
½ tsp fenugreek seeds	1 tsp allspice
½ tsp cardamom seeds	2 tbsp cayenne pepper
½ tsp coriander seeds	2 tbsp paprika
½ tsp ajowan seeds	1 tsp sea salt

Toast the whole spices in a dry frying pan over a low heat for about 2 minutes,
shaking the pan to ensure they don't burn, until they start to brown and release
their aroma. Remove from the heat immediately and leave to cool, then grind to
a powder using a pestle and mortar or grinder. Stir in the cayenne, paprika and
salt and grind again. Store in an airtight container out of direct sunlight.

Berbere paste: mix all the ground spices with 3 finely chopped garlic cloves,
1 tablespoon of grated root ginger, 3 tablespoons of vegetable oil and
2 tablespoons of red wine. Store in a sealed jar in the refrigerator.

NUTRIENT BALANCE (per portion)
14% protein, 32% fat, 40% carbohydrate, 14% fibre

VITAMINS AND MINERALS (percentage of RDA)
Vitamin A 23%, B1 2%, B2 3%, B3 3%, potassium 4%, calcium 2%, magnesium 2%, iron 10%,
zinc 1%, copper 3%, manganese 9%

HEALTH BENEFITS
Stimulates metabolism, circulation and immunity | improves digestion | encourages body to
burn fat

Tsire

Tsire is a typical West African spice mix made with peanuts. It can be used as a rub-on seasoning for grilling/broiling, to flavour sauces, as a condiment, or spread on toast like peanut butter.

Preparation and cooking time: 10 minutes, plus cooling

To fill a 100ml/3½fl oz jar

100g/3½oz/¾ cup peanuts

1 tbsp dried chilli/hot pepper flakes or chilli powder

8 whole cloves

5cm/2in cinnamon stick, broken up

½ tsp ground ginger

½ tsp freshly grated nutmeg

½ tsp sea salt

Toast the peanuts, chilli, cloves and cinnamon in a dry frying pan over a low heat, shaking the pan to ensure they don't burn, until they start to brown and release their aroma. Remove from the heat immediately and leave to cool, then grind coarsely using a pestle and mortar or grinder. Store in an airtight container in a cool, dry place for about 6 weeks.

Variation: To season food for grilling/broiling or baking, add a little oil to the tsire to form a paste and spread over meat, fish or vegetables.

NUTRIENT BALANCE (per portion)
18% protein, 64% fat, 12% carbohydrate, 6% fibre

VITAMINS AND MINERALS (percentage of RDA)
Vitamin A 7%, E 9%, B1 12%, B2 2%, B3 10%, B5 5%, B6 5%, folate 6%, biotin 15%, potassium 6%, calcium 4%, magnesium 8%, iron 8%, zinc 5%, copper 13%, manganese 24%, selenium 1%, iodine 1%

HEALTH BENEFITS
High in monounsataturated fat and antioxidants | may help lower the risk of cardiovascular disease and cancer | warming and stimulating

Ras El Hanout

Ras el hanout is Arabic for 'head of the shop', and in this context it means the best spice blend available, or the king of spice blends. It originated in Morocco and is used all over North Africa in savoury dishes: as a rub-on seasoning before grilling/broiling or frying, and stirred into couscous and rice. Ras el hanout always contains a long list of spices that varies from one kitchen to the next. Here is a typical blend.

Preparation and cooking time: 10 minutes, plus cooling

To fill a 100ml/3½fl oz jar

½ tsp cayenne pepper

1 tsp coriander seeds

1 tsp cumin seeds

½ tsp black peppercorns

2.5cm/1in cinnamon stick, broken up

½ tsp fenugreek seeds

½ tsp whole cloves

1 tsp cardamom seeds, from green
    cardamom pods

4 tbsp paprika

2 tsp ground turmeric

Toast the spices in a dry frying pan over a low heat, for 1–2 minutes, shaking the pan to ensure they don't burn, until they start to brown and release their aroma. Remove from the heat immediately and leave to cool, then grind to a powder using a pestle and mortar or grinder. Store in an airtight container in a cool, dry, dark place for up to 6 months.

Variations: Try adding any of the following: melegueta pepper, rose hips, galangal root, allspice, nutmeg or ground ginger to create a unique blend of your own.

NUTRIENT BALANCE (per portion)
15% protein, 31% fat, 40% carbohydrate, 14% fibre

VITAMINS AND MINERALS (percentage of RDA)
Vitamin A 24%, B1 2%, B2 4%, B3 3%, potassium 5%, calcium 2%, magnesium 3%, iron 11%, zinc 2%, copper 4%, manganese 6%

HEALTH BENEFITS
Stimulates circulation and digestion | warming and healing | encourages body to burn fat

Piri Piri Sauce

Also known as peri peri and pili pili, *piri piri* is Swahili for 'pepper pepper', referring to a very hot sauce made with red chillies. The name is used in those parts of Africa that had a Portuguese influence, and it is thought that the Portuguese brought chillies to their African colonies from South Africa. Piri piri sauce is versatile, and can be used as a rub-on seasoning before grilling/broiling; to add spice to stews and casseroles; and as a condiment.

Preparation time: 10 minutes

Makes 200ml/7fl oz/scant 1 cup

8 red chillies, roughly chopped

2 tsp paprika

2 tsp coriander

4 garlic cloves, roughly chopped

1 tsp sea salt

1 tsp black peppercorns

juice of 2½ limes

100ml/3½fl oz/scant ½ cup olive oil

Put all the ingredients in a food processor or blender and blend to form a coarse sauce. Store in an airtight container in a cool, dark place for up to 4 weeks.

NUTRIENT BALANCE (per portion)
3% protein, 90% fat, 5% carbohydrate, 2% fibre

VITAMINS AND MINERALS (percentage of RDA)
Vitamin A 7%, E 2%, C 13%

HEALTH BENEFITS
Strongly antioxidant | antibiotic | immune system booster | stimulates circulation

Harissa

This Tunisian chilli sauce contains hot chillies, garlic and coriander and cumin seeds. It is used to flavour couscous and soups, as a dip or a side dish, and as a marinade for grilling/broiling. It is also popular for breakfast spread on toast or a flatbread. Recipes vary from household to household and from region to region, but here is the one that I prefer to use.

Preparation and cooking time: 15 minutes, plus cooling

To fill a100ml/3½fl oz jar

2 tbsp coriander seeds

1 tbsp cumin seeds

1 tsp caraway seeds

10 hot red chillies, roughly chopped

5 garlic cloves, roughly chopped

1 tsp sea salt

5 tbsp olive oil

Toast the seeds in a dry frying pan over a low heat for 1–2 minutes, shaking the pan to ensure they don't burn, until they start to brown and release their aroma. Remove from the heat immediately and leave to cool, then grind to a powder using a pestle and mortar or grinder. Transfer to food processor or blender with the remaining ingredients and whizz to a coarse paste. Store in an airtight container in the refrigerator for up to 3 weeks.

Variations: Try adding some lemon juice or, for a less hot version, use grilled/broiled red peppers in place of some of the chillies.

NUTRIENT BALANCE (per portion)
7% protein, 78% fat, 10% carbohydrate, 6% fibre

VITAMINS AND MINERALS (percentage of RDA)
Vitamin A 4%, E 2%, C 13%, B1 2% potassium 4%, calcium 4%, magnesium 5%, iron 10%, zinc 2%, copper 6%, manganese 6%

HEALTH BENEFITS
Stimulates heart, circulation and metabolism | antioxidant and antiseptic | may ease colic, digestive cramps and wind

Garam Masala

In Hindi, *garam* means 'hot/intense', and *masala* means 'spices', and garam masala ground spice blends are key to Indian cuisine. There is no definitive recipe. Ingredients change from region to region and from cook to cook, but here is my personal favourite.

Preparation time: 5 minutes

To fill a100ml/3½fl oz jar

3 tbsp cardamom seeds

5cm/2in cinnamon stick

2 tsp cumin seeds

½ tsp black peppercorns

3 whole cloves

1 bay leaf

½ tsp freshly grated nutmeg

1 star anise

Put all the spices in a pestle and mortar or grinder and grind to make a powder. Store in an airtight container until needed.

Variations: Try adding white peppercorns, black cumin and black, brown or green cardamoms. You can also add nuts, garlic or onion, and a little water, vinegar or coconut milk to make garam masala paste.

NUTRIENT BALANCE (per portion)
12% protein, 24% fat, 44% carbohydrate, 19% fibre

VITAMINS AND MINERALS (percentage of RDA)
Potassium 3%, calcium 3%, magnesium 3%, iron 27%, copper 5%, manganese 18%

HEALTH BENEFITS
Antiseptic | soothes digestion | reduces inflammation | may inhibit cancer cell proliferation

Curry Powder

Curry powders are an essential feature of south Asian cooking. They tend to be hotter than garam masala blends but vary enormously as they are mixed to suit different dishes. Here is a Tamil curry powder, also called a sambar, which I particularly like.

Preparation and cooking time: 10 minutes, plus cooling

To fill a 50ml/1¾fl oz jar

2 tbsp coriander seeds

1 tbsp cumin seeds

1 tsp fenugreek seeds

1 tsp mustard seeds

3 whole cloves

½ tsp black peppercorns

1 cinnamon stick or 5cm/2in piece cassia

1 tsp cayenne pepper

½ tsp asafoetida

1 tsp ground turmeric

5cm/2in piece of jaggery (optional)

1 tsp sea salt

Toast all the seeds, cloves and cinnamon in a dry frying pan over a low heat for about 2 minutes, shaking the pan to ensure they don't burn, until they start to brown and release their aroma. Remove from the heat immediately and leave to cool. Grind to a powder with the remaining ingredients using a pestle and mortar or grinder. Store in an airtight container.

Variations: There are endless curry powder combinations: try creating mixtures adding ginger, garlic, paprika, fennel seeds, caraway, cardamom, nutmeg, celery seeds, bay leaf, tamarind or curry leaf in addition to the ingredients listed above.

NUTRIENT BALANCE (per portion)
16% protein, 36% fat, 33% carbohydrate, 16% fibre

VITAMINS AND MINERALS (percentage of RDA)
Vitamin A 2%, potassium 3%, calcium 4%, magnesium 3%, iron 8%, zinc 2%, copper 5%, manganese 7%

HEALTH BENEFITS
Calms digestion | promotes healthy bowel flora | improves blood sugar control | reduces blood cholesterol levels | immune boosting and anti-cancer

Panch Phoron

Panch phoron is a Bengali five-spice mixture consisting of whole seeds, and is used widely in Bangladesh and eastern India to flavour curries, dals and pickles. The blend is commonly used to flavour pulses and vegetable dishes.

Preparation time: 5 minutes

To fill a 50ml/1¾fl oz jar

1 tbsp nigella seeds

1 tbsp fenugreek seeds

1 tbsp cumin seeds

1 tbsp mustard seeds

1 tbsp fennel seeds

Mix the seeds together and store in an airtght container for 4–6 months.

To use, fry a measure of the mixture in hot oil until the seeds begin to pop, then stir in the rest of the ingredients in your recipe so that they become coated in the spices before continuing cooking.

Variation: Celery seeds can replace the mustard seeds.

NUTRIENT BALANCE (per portion)
21% protein, 41% fat, 28% carbohydrate, 10% fibre

VITAMINS AND MINERALS (percentage of RDA)
Vitamin B1 2%, B3 2%, potassium 3%, calcium 5%, magnesium 4%, iron 14%, zinc 2%, copper 6%, manganese 8%

HEALTH BENEFITS
Improves digestion | may help chronic health problems | may help cardiovascular disorders, cancer and allergy

Suwanda Kudu

Translated as 'fragrant mixture', suwanda kudu is a mild spice blend popular in Sri Lankan cuisine, especially for making pancakes, curries and chutneys.

Preparation and cooking time: 10 minutes, plus cooling

To fill a 50ml/1¾fl oz jar

1 cinnamon stick

5 whole cloves

1 tsp black cumin seeds

1 tsp coriander seeds

1 tsp nigella seeds

1 tsp cardamom seeds

½ tsp fenugreek seed

Toast the spices in a dry frying pan over a low heat for 1–2 minutes, shaking the pan so they don't burn, until they start to brown and release their aroma. Remove from the heat immediately and leave to cool, then grind to a powder using a pestle and mortar or grinder. Store in an airtight container.

Variations: Though slightly different in flavour, allspice is also sometimes referred to as suwanda kudu and can be used as a substitute in recipes.

NUTRIENT BALANCE (per portion)
15% protein, 32% fat, 34% carbohydrate, 19% fibre

VITAMINS AND MINERALS (percentage of RDA)
Potassium 3%, calcium 4%, magnesium 3%, iron 15%, zinc 2%, copper 5%, manganese 12%

HEALTH BENEFITS
Warming and stimulating | calms the digestion and relieves colic | antibiotic and antiviral | helps relieve arthritis | increases peripheral circulation | may help to reduce high blood pressure

Chinese Five Spice

Ngo-Hiong, or Chinese five spice, is a mild, distinctive mixture of five or six, or sometimes more, spices that gives a characteristic aniseedy taste to many Chinese and Asian dishes. It can also be mixed with salt and used as a condiment to serve with fried foods.

Preparation time: 5 minutes

To fill a 50ml/1¾fl oz jar
5cm/2in piece of cassia bark

12 whole cloves

2 tsp fennel seeds

2 tsp Szechuan peppercorns

3–4 star anise

Put all the ingredients in a pestle and mortar or grinder and grind to a powder. Store in an airtight container in a cool, dry place for up to 6 months.

Variations: Other combinations may contain aniseed, cardamom, liquorice, black pepper, galangal, ginger, nutmeg, turmeric, cinnamon or dried mandarin orange peel.

NUTRIENT BALANCE (per portion)
14% protein, 34% fat, 33% carbohydrate, 18% fibre

VITAMINS AND MINERALS (percentage of RDA)
Potassium 3%, calcium 5%, magnesium 3%, iron 7%, zinc 2%, copper 4%, manganese 15%

HEALTH BENEFITS
Simultaneously stimulating and calming | helps relieve colic and wind | antibiotic, antiviral and antioxidant | may help reduce the risk of developing cancer and cardiovascular disease

SNACKS AND LIGHT BITES

Olives De Picar

Spanish finger foods are called *cosas de picar*, or 'things to nibble', and include a variety of light dishes served as snacks or aperitifs. Marinated olives are a tapas favourite and very easy to prepare.

Preparation time: 5 minutes, plus marinating | Calories per portion: 92

Serves 4
100g/3½oz/¾ cup green olives
1 red chilli, finely sliced
3 garlic cloves, finely sliced
2 lemongrass stalks, peeled, trimmed and finely chopped
2 tbsp olive oil

Mix all the ingredients together in a bowl, cover and leave to marinate in the refrigerator for an hour or so before serving.

NUTRIENT BALANCE (per portion)
4% protein, 88% fat, 6% carbohydrate, 2% fibre

VITAMINS AND MINERALS (percentage of RDA)
Vitamin A 10%, E 10%, C 30%, folate 5%, potassium 8%, copper 8%, manganese 28%

HEALTH BENEFITS
High in monounsaturated oils and oleic acid | good for heart and circulation | may help reduce inflammation

Roasted Spiced Nut Mix

Use this spiced nut mixture to add some hot crunch to soups and salads, or serve simply as a snack.

Preparation and cooking time: 10 minutes | Calories per portion: 115

Serves 4

2 tbsp sunflower seeds

2 tbsp pine nuts

2 tbsp roughly chopped pecan nuts

3 tbsp soy sauce

1 tbsp lemon juice

2 tsp Piri Piri Sauce (see page 111)

Toast the seeds and nuts in a dry frying pan over a medium heat for 2 minutes, shaking the pan to ensure they don't burn, until they start to change colour. Add the remaining ingredients, turn the heat down and stir-fry until all the liquid has evaporated. Remove from the heat and cool completely before serving, or store in an airtight container.

Variations: Any mixture of nuts and seeds can be used for this recipe. Adjust the hotness by adding more or less of the piri piri. You can also replace the piri piri with Tabasco sauce.

NUTRIENT BALANCE (per portion)
10% protein, 80% fat, 7% carbohydrate, 3% fibre

VITAMINS AND MINERALS (percentage of RDA)
Vitamin E 46%, B1 28%, B2 5%, B3 8%, potassium 12%, magnesium 23%, iron 14%, zinc 17%, copper 48%, manganese 74%, selenium 11%

HEALTH BENEFITS
High in omega oils and antioxidants | good for skin, blood, bones, hair and nails

Spiced Figs

These little balls of energy are versatile and easy to make. Eat them as a snack, part of a finger-food buffet or as a festive treat.

Preparation and cooking time: 10 minutes | Calories per fig: 83

Makes 24

2 tbsp aniseeds

2 tbsp sesame seeds

24 dried figs

24 Brazil nuts

2 tbsp unsweetened cocoa powder

Toast the seeds in a small, dry frying pan over a low heat, shaking the pan to ensure they don't burn, until they start to brown and release their aroma. Leave to cool for a few minutes, then grind to a fine powder using a pestle and mortar or grinder.

Slice each fig almost through horizontally from the fat end, open it and fill with a pinch of the seed mixture and a Brazil nut. Close up the fig and dip it in the cocoa powder. Repeat the process with the remaining ingredients, then serve.

NUTRIENT BALANCE (per portion)
8% protein, 32% fat, 53% carbohydrate, 7% fibre

VITAMINS AND MINERALS (percentage of RDA)
Potassium 12%, calcium 9%, magnesium 9%, iron 11%, manganese 9%, selenium 11%

HEALTH BENEFITS
Low calorie | aids digestion | good for skin, blood, hair and nails

Celery Seed Crackers

Preparation and cooking time: 30 minutes | Calories per cracker: 101

Makes 24

2 tsp celery seeds

1 tsp sea salt

4 tbsp rolled oats

4 tbsp sesame seeds

4 tbsp flaxseeds

4 tbsp sunflower seeds

4 tbsp pumpkin seeds

200g/7oz/1½ cups spelt flour

1 tsp baking powder

4 tbsp olive oil

Crush the celery seeds with the salt using a pestle and mortar or grinder, then tip into a large bowl and mix together with the remaining dry ingredients. Add 100ml/3½fl oz/scant ½ cup water and the oil and mix well to form a smooth, slightly sticky dough.

Preheat the oven to 200°C/400°F/Gas 6. Lay a sheet of baking parchment (to fit a baking sheet) onto a flat surface, put the dough onto it and cover with another sheet of baking parchment Roll out the dough between the parchment sheets, using a rolling pin, until about 5mm/¼in thick. Transfer to the baking sheet, still in the paper. Remove the top sheet of paper, prick the dough all over with a fork and score into cracker-size squares. Bake for about 15 minutes, or until the crackers look crisp and golden. Leave to cool on a wire/cooling rack before serving.

NUTRIENT BALANCE (per portion)
14% protein, 52% fat, 29% carbohydrate, 5% fibre

VITAMINS AND MINERALS (percentage of RDA)
Vitamin E 9%, B1 10%, B3 5%, calcium 5%, magnesium 12%, iron 9%, zinc 8%, copper 18%, manganese 30%, selenium 13%

HEALTH BENEFITS
Low calorie | blood cleansing | immune system booster

Spiced Hummus

Hummus is a perfect dip to serve with raw vegetables or breadsticks. The addition of jalapeño peppers provides extra heat to the dish.

Preparation time: 10 minutes | Calories per portion: 122

Serves 6

400g/14oz chickpeas, drained and rinsed

2 garlic cloves, crushed

1 tsp ground cumin

2 jalapeño peppers, finely chopped

100ml/3½fl oz/scant ½ cup lemon juice

1 tsp sea salt

2 tbsp tahini

Put all the ingredients, except the tahini, and 100ml/3½fl oz/scant ½ cup water in a food processor or blender and blend to a smooth paste. Stir in the tahini and mix well. Adjust the seasoning, if necessary.

Serve with raw vegetable sticks, breadsticks or pitta bread, if you like.

Tip: For a milder blend, remove all the seeds from the jalapeños to reduce their heat.

NUTRIENT BALANCE (per portion)
17% protein, 30% fat, 46% carbohydrate, 6% fibre

VITAMINS AND MINERALS (percentage of RDA)
Vitamin C 16%, B1 9%, B5 6%, B6 30%, folate 28%, potassium 12%, calcium 9%, magnesium 13%, iron 18%, zinc 11%, copper 23%, manganese 28%

HEALTH BENEFITS
High in protein and unsaturated fats | good for circulation | stimulates digestion

Spicy Tuna Dip

Preparation time: 5 minutes | Calories per portion: 154

Serves 4

200g/7oz canned tuna, drained (or tofu, crumbled)

¼ red onion, finely chopped

3 tbsp mayonnaise

3 tbsp plain soy yogurt

2 tbsp capers

1 tbsp paprika, plus extra to serve

½ tsp ground Szechuan pepper

1 tbsp lemon juice

sea salt, to taste

Mix all the ingredients together in a bowl. Transfer to a serving dish and sprinkle with a little extra paprika. Cover and chill in the refrigerator until ready to serve.

Serve with Celery Seed Crackers (see page 123), tortilla chips or pitta bread, if you like.

Variation: Use freshly ground black pepper as a substitute if Szechuan pepper is not available.

NUTRIENT BALANCE (per portion)
34% protein, 61% fat, 5% carbohydrate, 1% fibre

VITAMINS AND MINERALS (percentage of RDA)
Vitamin E 21%, B3 19%, B6 9%, B12 28%, potassium 8%, magnesium 6%, iron 6%, copper 7%, selenium 60%, iodine 3%

HEALTH BENEFITS
Rich in omega-3 oils | good for skin, hair, nails, heart, circulation and blood

Sushi Rolls

My seven-year-old daughter adores *hosomaki* (small sushi rolls) with avocado filling and can easily eat 16 all by herself, given half a chance. An easy, healthy snack, or a meal in itself served with steamed, lightly salted, green soy beans (edamame beans).

Preparation and cooking time: 30 minutes, plus chilling | Calories per portion: 454

Serves 4

250g/9oz/1⅓ cups sushi rice

2 tbsp mirin or rice vinegar

1 package sushi nori sheets

1 avocado, peeled, pitted and cut into long, thin strips

125g/4½oz fresh tuna steak, cut into long, thin strips

125g/4½oz smoked tofu, cut into long thin, strips

½ cucumber, cut into long, thin strips

5 spring onions/scallions, cut into long, thin strips

1 carrot, peeled, cut into long, thin strips

sea salt

Rinse the rice under cold running water. Drain and pour into a saucepan with 500ml/17fl oz/2 cups water and a pinch of salt. Bring to the boil, cover and leave to simmer for 15–20 minutes until the water is absorbed. Remove the rice from the heat and leave to one side for a few minutes, then tip into a large, flat dish and mix in the mirin. Prepare the filling ingredients while the rice is cooking and cooling.

Use a bamboo sushi mat to help roll the *maki*. First, put a sheet of nori on the mat. Dip your fingers in cold water, then spread the rice over three-quarters of the seaweed in an even, 5mm/¼in thick layer, leaving the quarter furthest away clear. Put some filling ingredients (either one type or in combinations, as you prefer) in a line across the rice, from left to right. Wet the far edge of the nori, then roll up the bamboo mat slowly away from yourself, tucking in the nearer edge of the sushi roll and pressing gently with both hands as you roll to the far edge. Transfer the roll from the bamboo mat to a tray, with the joined edge downward. Repeat with the remaining ingredients, then cover in cling film/plastic wrap and chill in the refrigerator until ready to serve.

Before serving, use a lightly moistened sharp knife to trim the ends, then cut each roll into 8 pieces. Discard the end pieces, then transfer the rolls to a large serving tray, cut side up.

Serve with pickled ginger, wasabi paste and little bowls of soy sauce, if you like.

Variations: Leave out the mirin and the tuna steak, if you prefer. For a spicier version, smear a thin layer of wasabi on the rice before you add the filling.

NUTRIENT BALANCE (per portion)
22% protein, 26% fat, 45% carbohydrate, 8% fibre

VITAMINS AND MINERALS (percentage of RDA)
Vitamin A 124%, D 43%, E 14%, C 29%, B1 25%, B2 40%, B3 49%, B5 17%, B6 31%, folate 28%, biotin 4%, potassium 56%, calcium 27%, magnesium 22%, iron 33%, zinc 33%, copper 59%, manganese 88%, selenium 42%, iodine 76%

HEALTH BENEFITS
Protein and micronutrient rich | stimulates metabolism | helps maintain energy levels | good for eyes, skin, cell repair and general immunity

African Seafood Brochettes

For a vegetarian alternative, substitute tofu for the large prawns/jumbo shrimp.

Preparation and cooking time: 30 minutes | Calories per portion: 290

Serves 4

20 raw, large prawns/jumbo shrimp, peeled and deveined (or 250g/9oz tofu, cubed)

4 sheets of nori seaweed, cut into small squares

1 sweet potato, quartered and cut into thin chunks

2 red onions, quartered

20 okra, halved

1 green pepper, deseeded and cut into chunks

20 cherry tomatoes

20 button mushrooms

2 tbsp olive oil

100ml/3½fl oz/scant ½ cup Tsire (see page 109)

Spear the prawns/shrimp, nori and vegetables onto barbecue skewers in an alternating pattern. Pour the oil into a bowl, add the tsire and stir well, then brush the brochettes with the mixture. Cook on a hot barbecue or under a preheated hot grill/broiler, and cook until the prawns/shrimp turn pink and the vegetables are cooked through and golden, brushing with more of the tsire oil as you turn them.

Variations: Try Piri Piri Sauce (see page 111) in place of the tsire.

NUTRIENT BALANCE (per portion)
27% protein, 48% fat, 20% carbohydrate, 5% fibre

VITAMINS AND MINERALS (percentage of RDA)
Vitamin A 44%, E 36%, C 33%, B1 38%, B2 28%, B3 35%, B5 25%, B6 27%, folate 34%, biotin 28%, potassium 51%, calcium 23%, magnesium 30%, iron 33%, zinc 27%, copper 67%, manganese 59%, selenium 39%, iodine 36%

HEALTH BENEFITS
High in protein, micronutrients and antioxidants | good energy booster

Paprika Latkes with Prawn Mayonnaise

The secret to making crispy latkes, or potato pancakes, is to use a dry, floury potato variety, such as King Edward or russet. For a vegetarian alternative, substitute the prawns/shrimp with cashew nuts.

Preparation and cooking time: 30 minutes | Calories per portion: 492

Serves 4

For the potato cakes

3 large baking potatoes, coarsely grated

1 tbsp sweet paprika

olive oil, for frying

sea salt and freshly ground black pepper

For the prawn mayonnaise

250g/9oz cooked peeled prawns/shrimp (or 100g/3½oz cashew nuts)

4 tbsp mayonnaise

1 tbsp chopped dill

1 tbsp lemon zest

2 tbsp finely chopped almonds

soy sauce

Put the grated potatoes in a sieve/strainer or colander and squeeze out the moisture. Transfer to a bowl and mix in the paprika, salt and pepper.

Turn the prawns/shrimp in the mayonnaise, then add the dill and lemon zest. Toast the almonds in a dry frying pan, shaking the pan to ensure they don't burn, until golden. Add a dash of soy sauce at the end.

Heat a little oil in a large frying pan, add several spoonfuls of the potato mixture, pressing them flat with a spatula and fry until golden for 2–3 minutes on each side. Repeat with the remaining mixture.

Serve the latkes on a bed of lettuce or salad leaves/greens, if you like, and top each one with a spoonful of the prawn/shrimp mayonnaise and a sprinkle of almonds.

NUTRIENT BALANCE (per portion)

19% protein, 37% fat, 41% carbohydrate, 2% fibre

VITAMINS AND MINERALS (percentage of RDA)

Vitamin A 30%, E 39%, C 41%, B1 62%, B2 18%, B3 19%, B5 15%, B6 68%, folate 40%, biotin 12%, potassium 70%, calcium 17%, magnesium 30%, iron 22%, zinc 27%, copper 48%, manganese 25%, selenium 33%, iodine 22%

HEALTH BENEFITS

Provides a steady release of energy | antioxidant | stimulates the immune system

Spicy Welsh Rarebit Tartlets

Preparation and cooking time: 30 minutes, plus chilling | Calories per portion: 589

Serves 4

200g/7oz/1½ cups plain/all-purpose flour, plus extra for dusting

a pinch of sea salt

100g/3½oz vegetable margarine, diced

½ tsp curry powder

1 tsp poppy seeds

250g/9oz Cheddar or soy cheese, grated

200ml/7fl oz/scant 1 cup pale ale

1 tsp English mustard

½ tsp pink or black peppercorns

Preheat the oven to 180°C/350°F/Gas 4. Sift the flour and salt into a bowl and add the margarine, chopping it into the flour with a knife until it forms small lumps. Continue to rub in the fat and flour until the mixture resembles fine breadcrumbs. Add the curry powder, poppy seeds and 2–3 tablespoons cold water to make a firm dough. Roll into a ball, wrap in cling film/plastic wrap and chill for about 30 minutes.

Dust a work surface with a little flour, then roll out the dough thinly. Divide into 4, then press into four 11cm/4in tartlet pans. Prick the bottoms with a fork and bake blind for 8 minutes, or until golden and crisp.

Meanwhile, heat the remaining ingredients in a saucepan over a medium-low heat, stirring constantly until the mixture is smooth and runny. Pour the rarebit into each of the pastry cases/shells and brown under a preheated hot grill/broiler for a few minutes.

NUTRIENT BALANCE (per portion)
12% protein, 60% fat, 25% carbohydrate, 1% fibre

VITAMINS AND MINERALS (percentage of RDA)
Vitamin A 25%, D 40%, B1 30%, B2 31%, B3 11%, B6 15%, B12 65%, folate 18%, potassium 11%, calcium 48%, magnesium 11%, iron 19%, zinc 16%, manganese 25%

HEALTH BENEFITS
Energy booster | vitamin and mineral rich | good for blood and bones

Artichokes Provençal

Serve as a first course with crusty French bread.

Preparation and cooking time: 50 minutes | Calories per portion: 119

Serves 4

4 artichokes, stems and tough outer leaves
removed

2 tbsp olive oil

1 tsp sea salt

1 tsp white peppercorns

4 garlic cloves, roughly sliced

½ lemon, with peel, sliced

1 lemongrass stalk

1 bay leaf

Stand the trimmed artichokes close together in a saucepan. Sprinkle with the remaining ingredients and add enough water to cover. Bring to a steady boil and cook for 25–40 minutes, depending on the size of the artichokes, until the water has almost evaporated and the artichokes are tender.

Remove the artichokes from the pan and drain well upside down. Strain the reduced cooking water and serve with the artichokes as a light dipping sauce.

Variation: Replace the lemongrass with kaffir lime leaves.

NUTRIENT BALANCE (per portion)
11% protein, 56% fat, 25% carbohydrate, 9% fibre

VITAMINS AND MINERALS (percentage of RDA)
Vitamin C 48%, B1 7%, B2 5%, B3 5%, B6 11%, folate 21%, potassium 19%, calcium 8%, magnesium 13%, iron 18%, zinc 7%, copper 27%, manganese 41%

HEALTH BENEFITS
Good for the liver | aids fat metabolism | antioxidant, antibiotic, anti-inflammatory and diuretic | may help lower blood cholesterol

Broad Beans and Tomatoes

Fresh young broad/fava beans make a perfect snack simply eaten raw, popped directly from their shells. In Greece they are served in a tomato sauce as *koukia yiachni*, a dish inspired by Turkish and Middle Eastern cuisine that makes a quick snack on its own, or a light first course or meal with a piece of flatbread.

Preparation and cooking time: 25 minutes | Calories per portion: 183

Serves 4

2 tbsp olive oil

1 bunch of spring onions/scallions, sliced

1 tbsp tomato purée/paste

1 tbsp chopped dill leaves

1 tsp ajowan seeds

1 tsp paprika

1 tsp white peppercorns, ground

1 tsp grated jaggery or raw cane sugar

200ml/7fl oz/scant 1 cup vegetable stock

500g/1lb 2oz broad/fava beans, shelled

sea salt

Heat the oil in a saucepan over a medium heat and sauté the spring onions/scallions for 5 minutes to soften. Stir in the tomato purée/paste, dill, spices and sugar and heat through. Add the stock and broad/fava beans and leave to simmer for 10 minutes until tender. Season with salt. Serve hot.

NUTRIENT BALANCE (per portion)
19% protein, 45% fat, 27% carbohydrate, 8% fibre

VITAMINS AND MINERALS (percentage of RDA)
Vitamin A 24%, E 10%, C 75%, B1 8%, B2 8%, B3 29%, B5 104%, B6 11%, folate 105%, biotin 7%, potassium 27%, magnesium 12%, iron 20%, zinc 15%

HEALTH BENEFITS
High protein, low carbohydrate | anti-stress | good source of folate | helps boost tissue healing and energy

Moroccan Ratatouille on Toast

This is a spicy version of the traditional French recipe, which originates from Provence. The name ratatouille comes from the French word *touiller*, meaning 'to toss', and the secret to cooking a good ratatouille is to prepare the ingredients separately and then toss them all together.

Preparation and cooking time: 50 minutes | Calories per portion: 305

Serves 4

2 red peppers

4 large ripe tomatoes

3 tbsp olive oil

1 aubergine/eggplant, cut into thick sticks

1 red onion, chopped

2 tsp Ras el Hanout (see page 110)

3 garlic cloves

1 tbsp red wine vinegar

1 tsp sugar

2 small courgettes/zucchini, sliced

sea salt and freshly ground black pepper

4 slices of country bread

Toast the peppers in a hot, dry frying pan or under a preheated hot grill/broiler until their skins blacken and char. Transfer to a bowl cover with cling film/plastic wrap and leave to cool, then peel off the skins and remove the stems and seeds. Slice the skinned peppers into thick strips.

Cut a small cross across the top of each tomato, then put them in a heatproof bowl and cover with boiling water. Leave to stand for 2–3 minutes, or until the skins split, then drain. Peel off and discard the skins. Cut into quarters and discard the seeds.

Heat 2 tablespoons of the oil in a large frying pan over a high heat. Fry the aubergine/eggplant pieces for 5 minutes on each side, or until golden and releasing some of the oil they have absorbed. Remove from the pan and leave to one side. Turn the heat down to medium, add the remaining oil and sauté the onion for 2 minutes. Add the ras el hanout and garlic, followed by the tomatoes, peppers and aubergine/eggplant. Heat through, then add the vinegar and sugar. Stir-fry for 5 minutes, then add the courgettes/zucchini. Leave to simmer for 10 minutes. Season with salt and pepper.

Meanwhile, toast the bread. Put a large spoonful of ratatouille on each slice and serve immediately.

Variations: Use Harissa (see page 112) or chilli sauce instead of ras el hanout.

NUTRIENT BALANCE (per portion)
12% protein, 38% fat, 44% carbohydrate, 6% fibre

VITAMINS AND MINERALS (percentage of RDA)
Vitamin A 49%, E 26%, C 212%, B1 39%, B2 9%, B3 24%, B5 15%, B6 52%, folate 62%, biotin 7%, potassium 56%, calcium 18%, magnesium 19%, iron 25%, zinc 15%, copper 16%, manganese 50%, selenium 75, iodine 5%

HEALTH BENEFITS
Good immunity booster | enhances resistance to infection | good for vision, skin and mucous membranes | helps maintain healthy blood and bones

Sundried Tomato, Caper and Olive Bruschetta

Preparation and cooking time: 10 minutes | Calories per portion: 266

Serves 4

50g/1¾oz capers
125g/4½oz sundried tomatoes in oil
125g/4½oz/1 cup black olives, pitted
1 red chilli
1 handful of parsley
1 small red onion
1 tsp celery seeds, crushed
1 tsp grated jaggery or raw cane sugar
sea salt and freshly ground black pepper
4 slices of ciabatta bread

Chop or grind all the ingredients, except the bread, with a little of the sundried tomato oil to a coarse consistency. Season with salt and pepper.

Toast the ciabatta slices, top with the tomato mixture and serve hot.

Variation: Deseed the chilli for a milder version.

NUTRIENT BALANCE (per portion)
16% protein, 23% fat, 56% carbohydrate, 6% fibre

VITAMINS AND MINERALS (percentage of RDA)
Vitamin A 14%, E 10%, C 59%, B1 29%, B2 15%, B3 25%, B5 15%, B6 17%, folate 28%, potassium 66%, calcium 21%, magnesium 25%, iron 41%, zinc 12%, copper 65%, manganese 52%, selenium 18%

HEALTH BENEFITS
High in unsaturated fats | good for heart, blood and cell respiration | antioxidant

Savoury Chickpea Pancakes

Popular in India and southern France, savoury chickpea pancakes are easy to make, delicious and vegan, as well as gluten- and dairy-free.

Preparation and cooking time: 20 minutes, plus standing | Calories per portion: 77

Makes 8 small pancakes

150g/5½oz/1¼ cups chickpea (or gram) flour, sifted

2 tsp grated fresh turmeric, or 1 tsp ground turmeric

3 garlic cloves, finely chopped

1 tsp ajowan seeds

½ tsp cayenne pepper, or 1 small chilli, chopped

1 tsp sea salt

1 handful of parsley, finely chopped

oil, for frying

Mix together all the dry ingredients in a bowl, then gradually mix in 250ml/9fl oz/ 1 cup water to make a smooth batter. Leave the mixture to stand in the refrigerator for 15 minutes. Mix well again just before using, adding a little more water if necessary to form a pouring consistency.

Heat a little oil in a large frying pan over a high heat. Pour 2–3 tablespoons of batter into the pan and cook for 1–2 minutes, turning each pancake over as it becomes firm and golden. Serve immediately, or keep warm while you cook the remaining batter.

Variations: Add chopped onion and green peas to the mixture. Vary the spicing by substituting ginger for turmeric, cumin or coriander in place of the ajowan seeds.

NUTRIENT BALANCE (per portion)
24% protein, 17% fat, 52% carbohydrate, 6% fibre

VITAMINS AND MINERALS (percentage of RDA)
Vitamin C 5%, B1 9%, B6 8%, folate 42%, potassium 12%, calcium 5%, magnesium 10%, iron 13%, zinc 6%, copper 19%, manganese 20%, selenium 5%

HEALTH BENEFITS
High in protein | stimulates circulation and metabolism | anti-inflammatory

Stuffed Parathas

These Indian-inspired, pan-fried breads are stuffed with a mixture of vegetables and spices. They are wonderful on their own, served with a yogurt dip or pickles, and are also excellent as part of a picnic or a buffet lunch.

Preparation and cooking time: 30 minutes | Calories per portion: 135

Makes 8

For the dough

125g/4½oz/1 cup wholemeal/whole-
   wheat flour
125g/4½oz/1 cup plain/all-purpose flour,
plus extra for dusting
½ tsp sea salt
2 tbsp coconut oil or vegetable margarine

For the filling

½ tsp ajowan seeds
½ tsp black cumin seeds
1 tsp grated root ginger
½ tsp garam masala

1 carrot, grated
oil, for frying
sea salt

To make the dough, combine the flours and salt in a bowl and add the fat, chopping it into the flour with a knife and spoon until it forms small lumps. Continue to rub in the fat and flour until the mixture resembles fine breadcrumbs. Add 150ml/5fl oz/ scant ⅔ cup cold water, a little at a time, and knead to make a soft ball. Cover with a clean damp cloth and leave to one side while you make the filling.

Crush the spices coarsely using a pestle and mortar or grinder, then stir in the carrot and add salt to taste.

Divide the dough into 8 balls and cover with cling film/plastic wrap. Take a ball and roll it out on a floured surface to form a circle about 9cm/3½in in diameter. Place a portion of the filling in the middle, bring the edges together to cover the stuffing completely, press and seal tightly. Roll out the filled dough to form a 15cm/6in circle. Repeat the process with the remaining balls of dough and filling mixture.

Heat a little oil in a heavy frying pan or griddle/grill pan until sizzling hot.
Cook the paratha until both sides are golden, flipping it over several times.
Keep warm wrapped in foil while you cook the remainder.

Variations: Try different fillings according to what vegetables you have available.
I suggest grated white radish, cauliflower and mashed potato or peas.

NUTRIENT BALANCE (per portion)
12% protein, 23% fat, 62% carbohydrate, 4% fibre

VITAMINS AND MINERALS (percentage of RDA)
Vitamin A 12%, B1 12%, B3 7%, B5 5%, B6 8%, folate 7%, biotin 5%, potassium 5%,
calcium 5%, magnesium 9%, iron 9%, copper 11%, manganese 31%

HEALTH BENEFITS
Stimulates digestion | aids circulation

SOUPS AND SALADS

Chervil Soup

Preparation and cooking time: 25 minutes | Calories per portion: 210

Serves 4

2 tbsp olive oil

1 onion, finely chopped

1 leek, finely sliced

1 garlic clove, finely chopped

2 carrots, finely sliced

2 celery stalks, finely sliced

500g/1lb 2oz asparagus, chopped and
   tough ends removed

100ml/3½fl oz/scant ½ cup coconut or
   almond cream

1 handful of chervil, finely chopped

1 tsp ground white pepper

1 tsp sea salt

Heat the oil in a large saucepan over a medium heat. Add the onion, leek, garlic, carrots and celery and sauté for 5 minutes. Add the asparagus and 1l/35fl oz/ 4¼ cups boiling water. Bring to the boil, then turn the heat down to low, cover and leave to simmer for 5 minutes, or until the vegetables are tender but not soft. Stir in the cream and chervil. Heat through, season if necessary, and serve hot.

NUTRIENT BALANCE (per portion)
19% protein, 47% fat, 27% carbohydrate, 7% fibre

VITAMINS AND MINERALS (percentage of RDA)
Vitamin A 75%, E 18%, C 33%, B1 35%, B2 7%, B3 11%, B5 7%, B6 40%, folate 127%, potassium 61%, calcium 30%, magnesium 14%, iron 47%, zinc 23%, copper 25%, manganese 46%, selenium 5%

HEALTH BENEFITS
Blood cleansing | healing and nourishing | gentle diuretic

Hot Pumpkin Soup

Hokkaido pumpkins have a wonderful flavour, but can be substituted with squash or other pumpkin varieties.

Preparation and cooking time: 25 minutes | Calories per portion: 219

Serves 4

1 tbsp olive oil

1 small red onion, chopped

4 garlic cloves, chopped

1cm/½in piece of root ginger, peeled and chopped

½ tsp cayenne pepper

1 tsp sweet paprika

1 tsp ground coriander

1 hokkaido pumpkin, peeled, deseeded and cubed

2 sweet potatoes, diced

1.5l/52fl oz/6½ cups vegetable stock

200ml/7fl oz/scant 1 cup coconut milk

sea salt and freshly ground black pepper

Heat the oil in a large saucepan. Add the onion and sauté for 1 minute. Stir in the garlic, ginger and other spices and let them sizzle for a further minute, then add the pumpkin and sweet potatoes. Stir well so the vegetables are covered in spices, then pour in the stock. Bring to the boil, then turn the heat down to low and leave to simmer for 10 minutes, or until the vegetables are soft. Cool slightly, then pour into a blender and blend until smooth. Return to the pan and stir in the coconut milk. Heat through, season to taste and serve.

NUTRIENT BALANCE (per portion)
9% protein, 60% fat, 28% carbohydrate, 3% fibre

VITAMINS AND MINERALS (percentage of RDA)
Vitamin A 60%, E 20%, C 49%, B1 40%, B3 7%, B5 18%, B6 13%, folate 19%, potassium 33%, calcium 12%, magnesium 16%, iron 26%, zinc 11%, copper 24%

HEALTH BENEFITS
Promotes good circulation | may help decrease risk of certain cancers

Tamarind Tomato Soup

This soup is substantial enough to eat as a light meal on its own. It can also be effective as a quick fix against colds and flu.

Preparation and cooking time: 35 minutes | Calories per portion: 225

Serves 4

1 tbsp coconut oil

2 shallots, chopped

2 garlic cloves, chopped

2 red chillies, deseeded and chopped

1 tsp ground cumin

1 tsp ground coriander

3cm/1¼in piece of galangal root, peeled and chopped

55g/2oz/¼ cup split red lentils, drained and rinsed

1kg/2lb 4oz tomatoes, chopped

500ml/17fl oz/2 cups vegetable stock

1 tbsp tamarind paste

1 tbsp crushed jaggery or raw cane sugar

1 handful of coriander/cilantro leaves, chopped

sea salt

4 tbsp plain soy yogurt, to serve (optional)

Heat the oil in a large saucepan over a medium heat. Add the shallots, garlic, chillies, cumin and ground coriander and leave to sizzle for 30 seconds, then stir in the galangal and lentils and cook for another minute. Add the tomatoes and stir well over a high heat until the tomatoes blend with the spices. Add the stock, tamarind and jaggery and bring to the boil, then turn the heat down to low and leave to simmer for 15–20 minutes, or until the lentils are tender.

Blend to a creamy consistency, then season with salt to taste. Scatter in the chopped coriander/cilantro leaves, then serve each portion with a swirl of yogurt, if you like.

Variations: You can use black cumin instead of ordinary cumin, and ginger in place of galangal. The coriander/cilantro leaves can be replaced with chives or parsley leaves.

NUTRIENT BALANCE (per portion)

17% protein, 28% fat, 49% carbohydrate, 6% fibre

VITAMINS AND MINERALS (percentage of RDA)

Vitamin A 41%, E 28%, C 103%, B1 33%, B2 9%, B3 22%, B5 14%, B6 41%, folate 35%, biotin 8%, potassium 60%, calcium 12%, magnesium 18%, iron 46%, zinc 12%, copper 26%, manganese 33%

HEALTH BENEFITS

Promotes cardiovascular health | stimulates the circulation | antibiotic | gently laxative and cooling

Harissa Soup

Preparation and cooking time: 35 minutes | Calories per portion: 303

Serves 6

1 tbsp olive oil

1 leek, sliced

1 large onion, diced

2 red chillies, sliced

3 garlic cloves, chopped

1 tsp ground coriander

½ tsp ground cumin

1 tsp caraway seeds

2 tsp paprika

1 carrot, diced

1 parsnip, diced

1 thick slice of celeriac, diced

400g/14oz canned mixed beans, drained
    and rinsed

400g/14oz canned chickpeas, drained
    and rinsed

400g/14oz/scant 1⅔ cups canned
    chopped tomatoes

200g/7oz green beans, chopped

2l/70fl oz/8½ cups vegetable stock

sea salt and freshly ground black pepper

1 handful of mint leaves, chopped

Heat the oil in a large saucepan. Add the leek and onion, heat through, then add the chillies, garlic and spices. Sauté over a medium heat for 5 minutes, stirring, then add all the root vegetables. Cook, stirring continuously, until all the vegetables are coated in spices. Add the mixed beans, chickpeas and tomatoes. Stir and heat through again, then add the green beans and stock. Bring to the boil, turn the heat down to low, cover and leave to simmer for 15 minutes, or until the root vegetables are tender. Season to taste and serve hot with a sprinkling of mint leaves.

NUTRIENT BALANCE (per portion)
22% protein, 17% fat, 50% carbohydrate, 12% fibre

VITAMINS AND MINERALS (percentage of RDA)
Vitamin A 50%, E 11%, C 70%, B1 47%, B2 17%, B3 18%, B5 13%, B6 42%, folate 146%, potassium 62%, calcium 21%, magnesium 31%, iron 54%, zinc 24%, copper 64%, manganese 80%, selenium 14%

HEALTH BENEFITS
Nourishing and healing | excellent during convalescence | helps raise energy levels

Jamaican Jerk Soup

Jamaican jerk is a cooking style in which meat, fish, shellfish or tofu is dry-rubbed or marinated with spices and then grilled/broiled or fried.

Preparation and cooking time: 40 minutes, plus marinating | Calories per portion: 293

Serves 4

400ml/14fl oz/1⅔ cups Jamaican Jerk
  Marinade (see page 107)
250g/9oz chicken breast fillet, sliced
  (or tofu, cubed)
1 tbsp olive oil
1 leek, sliced

500g/1lb 2oz potatoes, cubed
1 tsp fenugreek seeds
1.5l/52fl oz/6½ cups vegetable stock
250g/9oz garden peas
sea salt and white pepper

Put the chicken pieces in a non-reactive bowl and pour over the jerk mixture. Cover and leave to marinate in the refrigerator for at least 30 minutes. Heat the oil in a large saucepan. Add the leek and stir over a medium heat for 1 minute, then add the marinated chicken and sauté for a further 5 minutes, stirring well. Add the potatoes and fenugreek, and heat through, stirring continuously, until everything is well mixed. Pour in the stock and bring to the boil, then add the peas. Reduce the heat to low and leave to simmer for 15 minutes, or until the potatoes are soft and the chicken is cooked through. Season with salt and white pepper and serve hot.

NUTRIENT BALANCE (per portion)
24% protein, 32% fat, 39% carbohydrate, 5% fibre

VITAMINS AND MINERALS (percentage of RDA)
Vitamin A 8%, E 6%, C 66%, B1 52%, B2 14%, B3 14%, B5 11%, B6 65%, folate 57%, potassium 42%, calcium 56%, magnesium 22%, iron 28%, zinc 22%, copper 50%, manganese 63%, selenium 24%

HEALTH BENEFITS
High in protein | energy booster | good for blood, bones and nerves

Caldo Verde

Caldo verde is a traditional Portuguese green cabbage soup that works equally well using kale or spring/collard greens. The addition of the smoked sausage, which can be pork, vegetarian or spicy chorizo, gives the soup an authentic flavour.

Preparation and cooking time: 30 minutes | Calories per portion: 307

Serves 6

2 tbsp olive oil, plus extra for frying

1 large onion, sliced

500g/1lb 2oz salad potatoes, sliced

1–2 tbsp mustard seeds

1 tbsp paprika

2l/70fl oz/8½ cups vegetable stock

500g/1lb 2oz green cabbage, spring/ collard greens or kale, shredded

250g/9oz smoked cocktail sausages, sliced

sea salt and freshly ground black pepper

Heat the oil gently in a large saucepan. Add the onion and potatoes and stir until they just start to soften. Add the spices, turn up the heat and sizzle for a minute or two, then pour in the stock. Bring to the boil, then turn down the heat and leave to simmer for 10 minutes, or until the potato slices have softened. Add the shredded greens and simmer for a further 5 minutes until tender. Season to taste.

Meanwhile, fry the sausage slices and scatter them into the soup just before serving.

NUTRIENT BALANCE (per portion)
16% protein, 56% fat, 25% carbohydrate, 3% fibre

VITAMINS AND MINERALS (percentage of RDA)
Vitamin A 70%, E 14%, C 134%, B1 23%, B2 11%, B3 12%, B5 7%, B6 45%, folate 65%, potassium 43%, calcium 20%, magnesium 20%, iron 28%, zinc 17%, manganese 47%, selenium 5%

HEALTH BENEFITS
Helps regulate metabolism | promotes tissue healing

Raw Beetroot Soup

This is a spicy, refreshing, no-cook soup that is filling and packed full of vitamins and flavour. Peppercorns from Madagascar are thought to have the finest flavour. Freshly crushed, they add a sharp and robust contrast to the earthy, sweet beetroot/beet flavour of the soup.

Preparation time: 20 minutes, plus chilling | Calories per portion: 182

Serves 4

2 tsp cumin seeds

1 cinnamon stick

1 tsp whole cloves

2 tsp black peppercorns

2 tbsp grapeseed oil

1kg/2lb 4oz raw beetroot/beet,
  finely chopped

1kg/2lb 4oz tomatoes, chopped

2 celery stalks, finely chopped

1 cucumber, peeled and finely chopped

4 tbsp plain yogurt, to serve

1 small handful of parsley, chopped

Crush the cumin seeds, cinnamon, cloves and peppercorns coarsely using a pestle and mortar or grinder. Put all the ingredients, including the spices, into a food processor or blender, and process until smooth. Add water to adjust the consistency, if required.

Serve the soup chilled, adding a swirl of yogurt and a sprinkling of chopped parsley to each serving.

NUTRIENT BALANCE (per portion)
23% protein, 32% fat, 45% carbohydrate, 10% fibre

VITAMINS AND MINERALS (percentage of RDA)
Vitamin A 30%, E 20%, C 72%, B1 20%, B3 13%, B5 13%, B6 22%, folate 155%, potassium 64%, calcium 15%, magnesium 13%, iron 39%, zinc 11%, copper 10%, manganese 84%

HEALTH BENEFITS
Stimulates cell respiration | good aid to slimming | helps the body make efficient use of energy

Tropical Salad

Preparation time: 15 minutes | Calories per portion: 435

Serves 4

2 avocados, peeled, pitted and cubed

1 mango, peeled, pitted and cubed

½ large onion, or 1 small red onion,
    finely sliced

1 large handful of spinach, shredded

1 tsp dried thyme

4 kaffir lime leaves, midvein removed,
    finely chopped

1 tsp peeled and finely chopped galangal

1 tbsp lime juice

2 tbsp olive oil

250g/9oz smoked salmon, sliced (or smoked
    tofu, cubed)

sea salt and freshly ground black pepper

Put all the ingredients, except the smoked salmon, into a large salad bowl and
gently mix everything together. Lay the smoked salmon pieces on top, season to taste
and serve.

NUTRIENT BALANCE (per portion)

18% protein, 51% fat, 26% carbohydrate, 5% fibre

VITAMINS AND MINERALS (percentage of RDA)

Vitamin A 179%, E 49%, C 113%, B1 28%, B2 28%, B3 48%, B5 30%, B6 60%, folate 61%,
biotin 5%, potassium 70%, calcium 27%, magnesium 30%, iron 31%, zinc 14%, copper 46%,
manganese 65%, selenium 26%

HEALTH BENEFITS

High in protein and unsaturated fats | stimulates the immune system | good for skin, bones,
muscles, hair and nails

Orange and Olive Tofu Salad

Preparation and cooking time: 20 minutes | Calories per portion: 104

Serves 4

4 oranges, peeled and sliced into rings

1 small red onion, finely chopped

1 handful of black olives, pitted

1 tsp ground cinnamon

½ tsp Szechuan peppercorns

2 tbsp olive oil

200g/7oz tofu, cubed

1 tbsp tamari or soy sauce

Put the oranges in a large salad bowl. Sprinkle over the onion, olives, cinnamon, peppercorns and 1 tablespoon of the oil.

Heat the remaining oil in a frying pan and fry the tofu for 5–10 minutes, turning regularly, until golden. Pour in the tamari, then remove the pan from the heat and stir to coat the tofu. Pour the tofu and sauce over the salad and serve.

Variations: This recipe also works well with cooked chicken pieces in place of the tofu, but ensure that they are cooked through (15–20 minutes). For a hotter version, add some grated ginger and use black peppercorns in place of Szechuan peppercorns.

NUTRIENT BALANCE (per portion)
20% protein, 28% fat, 44% carbohydrate, 8% fibre

VITAMINS AND MINERALS (percentage of RDA)
Vitamin E 5%, C 68%, B1 16%, B2 5%, B5 6%, B6 9%, folate 17%, potassium 15%, calcium 12%, magnesium 9%, iron 11%, zinc 5%, copper 21%, manganese 8%

HEALTH BENEFITS
High protein, low calorie | stimulates the immune system | provides quick energy

Waldorf Salad

This salad was first created at the Waldorf Hotel in New York City in the 1890s. The original recipe did not contain nuts, but most cookbooks written from the 1930s onward include walnuts.

Preparation and cooking time: 10 minutes | Calories per portion: 246

Serves 4

1 small green lettuce, shredded

1 sweet red apple, cored and diced

4 celery stalks, diced

1 small bunch of red seedless grapes, halved

4 tbsp mayonnaise or plain yogurt

1 tsp Dijon mustard

1 tsp paprika

1 tbsp olive oil

1 handful of walnuts

1 jalapeño pepper, diced

dash of soy sauce

Put a layer of shredded lettuce in a salad bowl, then add the diced apple, celery and grape halves.

Mix together the mayonnaise, mustard and paprika in a separate bowl, then pour over the salad. Toss well so all the ingredients are coated.

Heat the oil in a small frying pan and add the chopped walnuts and jalapeño. Stir-fry for a few seconds, add a little soy sauce, stir and remove from heat. Sprinkle the jalapeño and walnuts over the dressed salad and serve.

NUTRIENT BALANCE (per portion)
5% protein, 76% fat, 16% carbohydrate, 2% fibre

VITAMINS AND MINERALS (percentage of RDA)
Vitamin A 38%, E 28%, C 18%, B1 11%, B2 7%, B5 5%, B6 13%, folate 13%, potassium 15%, calcium 5%, magnesium 8%, iron 9%, zinc 5%, copper 21%, manganese 25%

HEALTH BENEFITS
High in omega-3 oils and flavonoids | stimulates circulation and immune system

Multi Kale Salad

Kale is a valuable winter leaf vegetable, packed with vitamins and minerals, and a surprisingly high level of protein, while being very low in calories. Combined with red cabbage, oranges and apricots in a sweet and spicy dressing, it makes a refreshing yet wholesome salad.

Preparation time: 10 minutes | Calories per portion: 204

Serves 4

2 large handfuls of curly kale, finely chopped

¼ red cabbage, finely shredded

2 oranges, peeled and sliced

10–15 dried apricots, chopped

150ml/5fl oz/scant ⅔ cup plain soy yogurt

1 tbsp Dijon mustard

1 tbsp grated horseradish

1 tsp honey or maple syrup

1 handful of cashew nuts

Mix together the chopped kale, red cabbage, oranges and apricots in a large salad bowl.

In a separate bowl, combine the yogurt with the mustard, horseradish and honey to form a thick dressing. Pour over the salad and toss gently. Sprinkle with the cashews and serve.

NUTRIENT BALANCE (per portion)
19% protein, 29% fat, 45% carbohydrate, 7% fibre

VITAMINS AND MINERALS (percentage of RDA)
Vitamin A 71%, E 22%, C 28%, B1 17%, B2 13%, B5 12%, B6 32%, folate 86%, potassium 62%, calcium 29%, magnesium 21%, iron 26%, zinc 11%, copper 29%, manganese 59%, selenium 13%

HEALTH BENEFITS
Helps lower blood cholesterol | may inhibit cancer cell growth | rich in antioxidants

MAIN COURSES

Moroccan Tagine

Preparation and cooking time: 50 minutes | Calories per portion: 510

Serves 4

2 tbsp olive oil

4 shallots, sliced

1 cinnamon stick

1 tsp ground cumin

1 tsp ground coriander

a pinch of saffron strands

½ tsp cayenne pepper

4 garlic cloves, crushed

400g/14oz chicken breast fillet (or seitan or
  tofu), cut into bite-size pieces

500g/1lb 2oz pumpkin, peeled, deseeded
  and cubed

500g/1lb 2oz sweet potatoes, peeled
  and cubed

400g/14oz canned chickpeas, drained
  and rinsed

1 tbsp tomato purée/paste

400ml/14fl oz/1⅔ cups red wine

500ml/17fl oz/2 cups vegetable stock

1 handful of dried apricots

sea salt and freshly ground black pepper

Heat the oil in a flameproof casserole dish or tagine. Add the shallots and sauté gently for 2 minutes. Stir in the spices and garlic and sizzle for 30 seconds before adding the chicken pieces, pumpkin, sweet potatoes and chickpeas. Stir-fry for 3 minutes, then add the tomato purée/paste, red wine, stock and apricots. Season with salt and pepper and bring to the boil, then turn the heat down, cover and leave to simmer gently for 30 minutes, or until the chicken is cooked through, the vegetables are very soft and the sauce has caramelized.

NUTRIENT BALANCE (per portion)
29% protein, 23% fat, 44% carbohydrate, 5% fibre

VITAMINS AND MINERALS (percentage of RDA)
Vitamin A 126%, E 27%, C 65%, B1 63%, B2 23%, B3 63%, B5 47%, B6 56%, folate 57%, biotin 5%, potassium 91%, calcium 20%, magnesium 33%, iron 55%, zinc 36%, copper 65%, manganese 97%, selenium 31%, iodine 6%

HEALTH BENEFITS
High in protein and micronutrients | low in saturated fats | strongly antioxidant | helps promote normal blood clotting | stimulates metabolism and circulation | improves regulation of blood sugar levels

Ethiopian Doro Wat

One of Ethiopia's most popular dishes, this stew traditionally includes boiled eggs, too, and is served with a large flatbread or *injera*, similar to an Indian chapati. Make this dish vegan by substituting seitan, tempeh, chickpeas or soy chunks for the chicken and use vegetable stock.

Preparation and cooking time: 50 minutes | Calories per portion: 390

Serves 4

2 tbsp Berbere spice mix (see page 108)

8 chicken drumsticks

4 tbsp olive oil

2 large onions, finely chopped

4 garlic cloves, crushed

2.5cm/1in piece of root ginger, peeled and grated

1 tbsp paprika

375ml/13fl oz/1½ cups chicken stock

sea salt

Rub the berbere spice mix into the chicken drumsticks so they are thoroughly coated. Heat the oil in a large, heavy sauté pan and cook the chicken for 5–7 minutes until golden. Add the onion and sauté for 5 minutes, until soft and golden. Stir in the garlic and ginger and cook for 1–2 minutes, then add the paprika. Pour in the stock, then turn the heat down to low and leave to simmer gently for 20–30 minutes, or until the chicken is cooked through and tender, stirring from time to time. Season with salt and serve hot.

NUTRIENT BALANCE (per portion)

29% protein, 62% fat, 7% carbohydrate, 1% fibre

VITAMINS AND MINERALS (percentage of RDA)

Vitamin A 34%, D 4%, E 8%, C 5%, B1 14%, B2 16%, B3 43%, B5 22%, B6 27%, folate 9%, biotin 8%, potassium 24%, calcium 8%, magnesium 12%, iron 23%, zinc 26%, copper 15%, manganese 7%, selenium 34%, iodine 7%

HEALTH BENEFITS

High in protein | low in saturated fat | immune system booster | antibiotic

Oriental Spiced Chicken Pie

Preparation and cooking time: 50 minutes | Calories per portion: 598

Serves 6

500g/1lb 2oz chicken breast fillet, cut into
  bite-size pieces

4 tbsp spelt or wholemeal/whole-wheat flour

2 tbsp coconut or vegetable oil, plus extra
  for greasing

5cm/2in piece of cassia bark

10 Szechuan peppercorns

10 curry leaves

1 onion, chopped

2.5cm/1in piece of root ginger, peeled and
  finely chopped

4 carrots, cut into thin sticks

1 large handful of green beans, sliced

1 tsp ground turmeric

400ml/14fl oz/1⅔ cups coconut milk

375g/13oz puff pastry dough

1 tbsp nigella seeds

sea salt and freshly ground black pepper

Roll the chicken pieces in the flour, season with salt and pepper and leave to
one side.

Preheat the oven to 200°C/400°F/Gas 6. Heat the oil gently in a large frying pan
or wok. Add the cassia, peppercorns, curry leaves, onion and ginger and gently
stir-fry until the onion is soft. Add the chicken pieces, reserving any remaining flour.
Turn up the heat and stir-fry until the pieces are golden all over. Add the carrots, green
beans and turmeric and mix together well. Stir-fry for another minute and then tip in
the reserved flour. Heat through, then stir in the coconut milk, turn the heat down to
low and leave to simmer for 10 minutes, stirring occasionally.

Meanwhile, grease a large ovenproof pie dish and roll out the pastry dough so it
is slightly larger than the dish, to make a lid for the pie. Spoon the stir-fried chicken
and vegetables into the dish and cover with the lid. Brush the top with a little water,
sprinkle with nigella seeds and cook in the middle of the oven for 25 minutes, or
until the pastry is puffed and golden. Serve hot.

Variation: For a vegetarian option, replace the chicken with seitan.

NUTRIENT BALANCE (per portion)

21% protein, 55% fat, 22% carbohydrate, 1% fibre

VITAMINS AND MINERALS (percentage of RDA)

Vitamin A 90%, D 2%, E 3%, C 9%, B1 26%, B2 12%, B3 56%, B5 23%, B6 33%, folate 27%, biotin 5%, potassium 31%, calcium 14%, magnesium 19%, iron 33%, zinc 18%, copper 34%, manganese 45%, selenium 21%, iodine 6%

HEALTH BENEFITS

Filling and nourishing | antioxidant | good for blood, bones, eyes and skin

Nordic Juniper Casserole

A contemporary version of a traditional Nordic casserole, this is especially good served with pearl spelt and redcurrant sauce.

Preparation and cooking time: 45 minutes | Calories per portion: 461

Serves 4

2 tbsp coconut or vegetable oil

500g/1lb 2oz pork fillet (or seitan or tempeh), cut into strips

6 juniper berries, crushed

500g/1lb 2oz mushrooms, sliced

4 garlic cloves, crushed

2 parsnips, chopped

3 tbsp soy sauce

2 tbsp spelt or wholemeal/whole-wheat flour

1 lovage sprig, chopped

200ml/7fl oz/scant 1 cup cream (almond, soy or dairy)

100ml/3½fl oz/scant ½ cup soy yogurt or crème fraîche

sea salt and freshly ground black pepper

Heat the oil in a flameproof casserole. Add the meat and juniper berries and brown over a high heat for 2 minutes. Add the mushrooms, garlic and parsnips and stir-fry for 5 minutes, then add the soy sauce and stir well. Turn the heat down and mix in the flour. Add the lovage and 100ml/3½fl oz/scant ½ cup water, stirring well to ensure there are no lumps. Gradually bring to the boil, then add the cream, turn the heat down to low and leave to simmer very gently for 20 minutes, or until the meat is tender and cooked through. Stir in the yogurt, season to taste and serve hot.

NUTRIENT BALANCE (per portion)
33% protein, 50% fat, 14% carbohydrate, 3% fibre

VITAMINS AND MINERALS (percentage of RDA)
Vitamin A 21%, D 16%, E 11%, C 15%, B1 158%, B2 65%, B3 79%, B5 80%, B6 69%, folate 53%, biotin 36%, potassium 64%, calcium 12%, magnesium 18%, iron 19%, zinc 30%, copper 106%, manganese 31%, selenium 55%, iodine 6%

HEALTH BENEFITS
High in protein and micronutrients | provides energy | strengthens body tissues

Hungarian Goulash

Preparation and cooking time: 1 hour 20 minutes | Calories per portion: 383

Serves 4

3 tbsp olive oil

2 onions, finely chopped

2 tbsp paprika

500g/1lb 2oz beef, cubed (or quorn or
   soy chunks)

2 garlic cloves, chopped

1 bay leaf

1 tsp caraway seeds, crushed

200g/7oz tomatoes, chopped

200ml/7fl oz/scant 1 cup vegetable stock

4 potatoes, diced

1 turnip, diced

4 carrots, diced

1 green pepper, deseeded and diced

sea salt and freshly ground black pepper

Heat the oil in a large, heavy saucepan. Add the onions and sauté until soft.
Remove the pan from the heat, add the paprika, then add the beef, garlic, bay
leaf and caraway and keep turning the mixture until the beef is completely coated.
Return the pan to the hob/stovetop, turn up the heat and brown the beef. Add the
tomatoes and stock and bring to the boil, then turn the heat down to low and leave
to simmer, half-covered, for 40 minutes, adding a little more water if necessary.
Add the vegetables and simmer for a further 20 minutes, until cooked through and
tender. Season to taste and serve hot.

NUTRIENT BALANCE (per portion)
35% protein, 37% fat, 25% carbohydrate, 4% fibre

VITAMINS AND MINERALS (percentage of RDA)
Vitamin A 195%, D 13%, E 15%, C 71%, B1 44%, B2 31%, B3 56%, B5 25%, B6 89%,
biotin 6%, folate 37%, potassium 64%, calcium 11%, magnesium 52%, iron 49%, zinc 60%,
copper 22%, manganese 25%, selenium 19%, iodine 12%

HEALTH BENEFITS
High in protein and micronutrients | good for eyes, blood, bones and skin

Szechuan Beef

Preparation and cooking time: 45 minutes, plus marinating | Calories per portion: 384

Serves 4

350g/12oz sirloin steak, cubed (or tempeh, cubed)

2 tbsp soy sauce

1 tbsp Szechuan peppercorns, crushed

2 tbsp coconut or vegetable oil

1 butternut squash, peeled, deseeded and cut into wedges

4 potatoes, scrubbed and cut into wedges

2 pears, cored and cut into wedges

4 garlic cloves, sliced

1 tbsp peeled and grated root ginger

2 tbsp rosemary

toasted sesame oil

sea salt

Preheat the oven to 200°C/400°F/Gas 6. Put the beef in a bowl with the soy sauce and Szechuan pepper and leave to marinate for at least 30 minutes. Pour half the coconut oil into a baking pan, then put in the oven to heat.

Put the butternut squash, potatoes and pear wedges in the baking pan and sprinkle over the garlic, ginger, rosemary, sesame oil and salt, then return to the oven for 30 minutes, or until the vegetables are soft.

Meanwhile, heat the remaining oil in a frying pan or wok. Add the marinated beef and stir-fry over a high heat for 3–5 minutes, or until the beef is brown but tender. Remove the beef from the pan, put on top of the cooked vegetables and serve.

NUTRIENT BALANCE (per portion)
27% protein, 34% fat, 35% carbohydrate, 4% fibre

VITAMINS AND MINERALS (percentage of RDA)
Vitamin A 152%, D 96%, E 34%, C 73%, B1 38%, B2 23%, B3 44%, B5 30%, B6 80%, B12 72%, folate 43%, biotin 4%, potassium 72%, calcium 20%, magnesium 32%, iron 32%, zinc 42%, copper 29%, manganese 29%, selenium 15%, iodine 9%

HEALTH BENEFITS
High in protein and micronutrients | aids healing and convalescence

Florence Fennel Bake

Cooking the fish on top of the finely sliced vegetables adds subtle flavour to this nourishing dish.

Preparation and cooking time: 45 minutes | Calories per portion: 271

Serves 4

500g/1lb 2oz potatoes, thinly sliced

1 large red onion, thinly sliced

4 beefsteak tomatoes, thinly sliced

1 fennel bulb, thinly sliced

4 thick white fish fillets

1 lemon, unpeeled, thinly sliced

1 handful of parsley, chopped

1 tbsp fennel seeds, lightly toasted
  and crushed

200ml/7fl oz/scant 1 cup vegetable
  stock

sea salt and freshly ground black pepper

Preheat the oven to 200°C/400°F/Gas 6. Grease a large ovenproof dish and cover the bottom with the potato slices. Season with salt and pepper, then add the onion, tomatoes and fennel slices in layers. Put the fish fillets on top, season well and cover with the lemon slices, parsley and fennel seeds. Pour in the stock, cover with foil and bake for 30 minutes, or until the fish starts to flake and the vegetables are soft. Serve hot.

Variation: For a vegetarian meal, replace the fish with 250g/9oz tofu.

NUTRIENT BALANCE (per portion)
30% protein, 21% fat, 43% carbohydrate, 6% fibre

VITAMINS AND MINERALS (percentage of RDA)
Vitamin A 31%, E 16%, C 110%, B1 52%, B2 12%, B3 30%, B5 24%, B6 75%, folate 64%, biotin 4%, potassium 69%, calcium 18%, magnesium 21%, iron 24%, zinc 17%, copper 31%, manganese 27%, selenium 20%, iodine 4%

HEALTH BENEFITS
Low calorie | antioxidant | anti-cancer | benefits digestion | good for blood, bones, hair, skin and nails

Citrus Chilli Sea Bass With Fennel and Potato Salad

The hot lemony marinade also works well with tofu, or any firm white-fleshed fish that you want to bake or grill/broil.

Preparation and cooking time: 30 minutes, plus marinating | Calories per portion: 407

Serves 6

1kg/2lb 4oz sea bass fillets

For the marinade

2 jalapeño peppers

3 garlic cloves

1 spring onion/scallion

6 tbsp lemon juice

½ tsp ground mace

sea salt and freshly ground black pepper

For the salad

1kg/2lb 4oz new potatoes, scrubbed

1 fennel bulb, sliced

1 bunch of red radishes, sliced

1 small bunch of dill, chopped

3 tbsp walnut oil

2 tbsp white wine vinegar

Preheat the oven to 200°C/400°F/Gas 6. Put the fish fillets in a non-reactive ovenproof dish. Put all the marinade ingredients in a food processor or blender and whizz together. Pour over the fish, turning the pieces to ensure they are well coated. Cover and leave to marinate in the refrigerator for 10 minutes. Bake the marinated fish for 20 minutes, or until tender.

Meanwhile, cook the potatoes in a pan of boiling water for about 15 minutes until just cooked. Drain and leave to cool a little, then transfer to a serving bowl and stir in the fennel, radishes and dill. Drizzle with the walnut oil and white wine vinegar, toss well and season with salt and pepper. Serve with the fish.

NUTRIENT BALANCE (per portion)

36% protein, 36% fat, 27% carbohydrate, 2% fibre

VITAMINS AND MINERALS (percentage of RDA)

Vitamin A 22%, E 5%, C 66%, B1 49%, B2 22%, B3 39%, B5 33%, B6 95%, folate 46%, biotin 1%, potassium 67%, calcium 13%, magnesium 25%, iron 15%, zinc 24%, copper 32%, manganese 20%, selenium 43%, iodine 4%

HEALTH BENEFITS

High protein | high in B vitamins and antioxidants | anti-cancer | good for digestion and circulation | helps build strong bones

Persian Biryani

Preparation and cooking time: 1 hour | Calories per portion: 614

Serves 4

1–2 tbsp coconut or vegetable oil

2 onions, chopped

1 handful of whole almonds

1 handful of cashew nuts

2 cardamoms

2 green chillies

½ tsp saffron strands

1 tsp black peppercorns

1 tsp cayenne pepper

2 tsp black cumin seeds

500g/1lb 2oz mushrooms, chopped

300g/10½ oz potatoes

350g/12oz/1¾ cups basmati rice

1 handful of dried apricots

2.5cm/1in piece of root ginger, peeled
   and finely chopped

4 garlic cloves, chopped

3 tbsp lemon juice

sea salt

Heat 1 tablespoon of the oil in a wok or large, heavy frying pan over a high heat. Add the onions, almonds and cashews and stir-fry until they just start to colour. Remove them from the pan and leave to one side. Grind all the spices together using a pestle and mortar or grinder.

Return the pan to the heat, adding a little more oil if necessary, and add the mushrooms, potatoes, the ground spices and a little salt. Add all the remaining ingredients and heat through, stirring continuously. Add 700ml/24fl oz/3 cups water to cover all the ingredients and bring to the boil. Turn the heat down, cover and leave to simmer gently for about 20 minutes, or until all the water is absorbed and the rice is cooked, adding a little more water if required. Return the cooked onion and nuts to the pan, heat through and serve hot.

Variation: For a meat version, substitute minced/ground beef for the mushrooms, browning it before adding the potatoes.

NUTRIENT BALANCE (per portion)

15% protein, 25% fat, 56% carbohydrate, 4% fibre

VITAMINS AND MINERALS (percentage of RDA)

Vitamin A 6%, E 24%, C 44%, B1 42%, B2 39%, B3 37%, B5 51%, B6 56%,
folate 54%, biotin 47%, potassium 64%, calcium 14%, magnesium 29%, iron 52%,
zinc 21%, copper 141%, manganese 61%, selenium 30%, iodine 6%

HEALTH BENEFITS

Provides energy | stimulates digestion, metabolism and circulation

Spicy Lentil Bake

Preparation and cooking time: 1½ hours | Calories per portion: 385

Serves 6

1 tbsp olive oil

1 onion, finely chopped

1 bay leaf

½ tsp ground cloves

1 tsp ground turmeric

1 tsp nigella seeds

4 garlic cloves, finely chopped

3 carrots, grated

2 celery stalks, finely sliced

250g/9oz/1¼ cups dried Puy lentils, rinsed

2 tbsp tomato purée/paste

1 tsp yeast extract, or 1 tbsp Worcestershire
    sauce

500ml/17fl oz/2 cups vegetable stock

1kg/2lb 4oz potatoes, peeled and chopped

3 tbsp vegetable margarine

100ml/3½fl oz/scant ½ cup soy milk

sea salt and freshly ground black pepper

Heat the oil in a saucepan over a medium heat. Add the onion, spices, garlic, carrots and celery and cook for 5 minutes until soft. Add the lentils and heat through. Add the tomato pureé/paste and yeast extract and stir-fry for a few more minutes. Pour in the stock and bring to the boil, then turn the heat down to low, cover and leave to simmer gently for 20 minutes. Remove the lid and simmer for a further 20 minutes until tender. Add more water or stock from time to time, if required.

Meanwhile, cook the potatoes in a pan of salted boiling water for 15 minutes, or until tender. Drain, then return to the pan and mash with the margarine and milk.

Preheat the oven to 180°C/350°F/Gas 4. Spoon the lentil mixture into a shallow ovenproof dish, top with the mashed potatoes and ruffle with a fork. Bake for 30 minutes, or until the top starts to turn golden and the filling bubbles through at the edges. Leave to stand for 5 minutes before serving.

Variation: For a meat version, substitute 500g/1lb 2oz minced/ground lamb for the lentils. Brown it in the oil after heating the spices, then stir in the vegetables and cook through as above.

NUTRIENT BALANCE (per portion)

18% protein, 20% fat, 57% carbohydrate, 5% fibre

VITAMINS AND MINERALS (percentage of RDA)

Vitamin A 72%, E 7%, C 31%, B1 58%, B2 23%, B3 19%, B5 13%, B6 90%, folate 67%, potassium 68%, calcium 11%, magnesium 25%, iron 49%, zinc 25%, copper 63%, manganese 56%, selenium 82%, iodine 5%

HEALTH BENEFITS

Provides steady energy release | helps protect against cell degeneration

Japanese Tofu Burgers

Preparation and cooking time: 25 minutes, plus cooling | Calories per portion: 301

Makes 8

1 tbsp olive oil, plus extra for frying

3 shallots, finely chopped

300g/10½oz shiitake or chestnut/cremini
   mushrooms, finely chopped

2 garlic cloves, finely chopped

250g/9oz firm smoked tofu, crumbled

2 tbsp wheatgerm

2 tbsp wholemeal/whole-wheat breadcrumbs

4 tbsp fine oat flakes

2 tbsp soy sauce

1 tsp ground sansho pepper

sea salt

8 burger buns

Heat 1 tablespoon of oil in a wok or frying pan over a medium heat. Gently sauté the shallots until soft, then add the mushrooms and garlic and stir-fry for 5 minutes until the mushrooms start to colour. Add the remaining ingredients and mix in just enough water to give a firm consistency. Season with a little salt if necessary and leave to cool.

Shape the cooled mixture into 8 burgers, pressing the mixture firmly into flat rounds. Heat a little oil in the frying pan and cook the burgers for about 3 minutes on each side until heated through.

Serve in the burger buns with the usual accompaniments, or as part of a Japanese style meal.

NUTRIENT BALANCE (per portion)
36% protein, 28% fat, 42% carbohydrate, 5% fibre

VITAMINS AND MINERALS (percentage of RDA)
Vitamin E 16%, C 7%, B1 43%, B2 34%, B3 29%, B5 5%, B6 48%, folate 33%, biotin 5%, potassium 26%, calcium 61%, magnesium 25%, iron 33%, zinc 29%, copper 37%, manganese 95%, selenium 22%

HEALTH BENEFITS
Anti-cancer | helps lower blood cholesterol | good for skin, bones and muscles

Stuffed Portobello Mushrooms

Preparation and cooking time: 30 minutes | Calories per portion: 427

Serves 4

8 large portobello mushrooms, cleaned

2 tomatoes, deseeded and chopped

8 tbsp grated Parmesan cheese or brewer's yeast flakes

2 slices of wholemeal/whole-wheat bread, crumbled

1 egg, or 1 tbsp olive oil

4 garlic cloves, finely chopped

1 tbsp flat leaf parsley, finely chopped

2 tbsp olive oil, plus extra for greasing

1 tsp sea salt

2 tsp Hot Peppercorn Mix (see page 106)

Preheat the oven to 200°C/400°F/Gas 6 and grease an ovenproof dish. Snap off and chop the mushroom stalks. Put them in a bowl and add the remaining ingredients. Mix everything together well. Using a teaspoon, scrape out and discard the gills from each mushroom. Put the mushroom caps upside down in the prepared ovenproof dish. Fill each mushroom with the stuffing mixture, sprinkle with a little oil and bake for 15 minutes, or until the tops are golden.

NUTRIENT BALANCE (per portion)
24% protein, 43% fat, 29% carbohydrate, 4% fibre

VITAMINS AND MINERALS (percentage of RDA)
Vitamin A 40%, D 12%, E 19%, C 44%, B1 35%, B2 64%, B3 53%, B5 51%, B6 34%, folate 51%, biotin 23%, potassium 62%, calcium 59%, magnesium 22%, iron 32%, zinc 39%, copper 77%, manganese 71%, selenium 43%, iodine 13%

HEALTH BENEFITS
Free from saturated fat and cholesterol | rich in micronutrients | antioxidant and immune system booster | good for heart and circulation

Thai Vegetable Curry

Preparation and cooking time: 1 hour | Calories per portion: 412

Serves 4

2 tbsp coconut or vegetable oil

1 small red onion, chopped

1 leek, thinly sliced

1 red pepper, finely chopped

1 red chilli, finely chopped

6 garlic cloves, finely chopped

1 tbsp peeled and grated root ginger

6 lemongrass stalks, peeled, trimmed and
  chopped

1 tbsp sweet paprika

2 tsp ground turmeric

1 tsp black cumin seeds

8 kaffir lime leaves, fresh or dried

1 carrot, diced

4 potatoes, diced

1 black radish, sliced

300ml/10½fl oz/1¼ cups vegetable stock

1 small head of broccoli, cut into florets

200g/7oz green beans, trimmed

200g/7oz baby sweetcorn

400ml/14fl oz/1⅔ cups coconut milk

1 large handful of coriander/cilantro leaves,
  chopped

sea salt

1 large handful of bean sprouts, rinsed,
  to serve

Heat the oil in a wok or a large frying pan over a medium heat. Add the onion, leek, red pepper, chilli, garlic and all the spices. Stir-fry for a few minutes until the onion has softened. Add the diced carrot, potatoes and radish. Heat through and add the stock. Bring to the boil, then turn the heat down to low, cover and leave to simmer for 10 minutes. Add the broccoli, green beans and baby sweetcorn and simmer for a further 5 minutes until the vegetables are tender but retain a little bite. Add the coconut milk and coriander/cilantro. Heat through, season to taste and serve sprinkled with bean sprouts.

Variations: Replace the black cumin with cumin; ginger with galangal; lemongrass and kaffir lime leaves with lemon zest or tamarind.

NUTRIENT BALANCE (per portion)

11% protein, 63% fat, 21% carbohydrate, 4% fibre

VITAMINS AND MINERALS (percentage of RDA)

Vitamin A 86%, E 12%, C 228%, B1 34%, B2 21%, B3 22%, B5 12%, B6 53%, folate 114%, biotin 1%, potassium 67%, calcium 17%, magnesium 34%, iron 67%, zinc 22%, copper 48%, manganese 100%, selenium 3%, iodine 2%

HEALTH BENEFITS

Nourishing and filling | antioxidant | helps maintain energy levels | good for heart, circulation, eyes, skin, nails and nerves

Gujarati Dal

Traditional Gujarati dal is a delicious sweet and sour dish often served at weddings in the Indian state of Gujarat.

Preparation and cooking time: 1 hour | Calories per portion: 425

Serves 4

3 tbsp coconut or vegetable oil

8 curry leaves

1 tsp ground coriander

1 tsp ground cumin

½ tsp cayenne pepper

1 tsp ground turmeric

1 green chilli, sliced

a pinch of asafoetida

250g/9oz/1¼ cups yellow split peas, rinsed and drained

1 ripe tomato, chopped

4 kokum slices

2 tbsp grated jaggery or raw cane sugar

1 tbsp tamarind paste

3 pitted dates, sliced

1 tsp amchoor

1 small handful of toasted peanut halves

2cm/¾in piece of root ginger, peeled and chopped

½ tsp mustard seeds

½ tsp fenugreek seeds

1 red chilli, chopped

3 whole cloves

1 cinnamon stick

1 bunch of coriander/cilantro leaves, chopped

350g/12oz/1¾ cups cooked basmati rice

sea salt

Heat 1 tablespoon of the oil in a large saucepan over a medium heat. Add the curry leaves, ground coriander, cumin, cayenne, turmeric, green chilli and asafoetida, stir and let them sizzle for 2 minutes. Tip in the split peas and 1l/35fl oz/4¼ cups water and bring to the boil, then turn the heat down and leave to simmer gently for 30 minutes. Stir in the tomato, kokum, jaggery, tamarind, dates, amchoor, peanuts and ginger and continue to simmer for a further 15 minutes. Season with salt to taste.

Meanwhile, heat the remaining oil in a small frying pan, add the mustard and fenugreek seeds, red chilli, cloves and cinnamon stick and let them sizzle for 2 minutes. Pour the hot spice mixture over the dal just before serving. Sprinkle over the coriander/cilantro leaves and serve hot with the cooked basmati rice.

NUTRIENT BALANCE (per portion)

19% protein, 29% fat, 43% carbohydrate, 9% fibre

VITAMINS AND MINERALS (percentage of RDA)

Vitamin A 38%, E 16%, C 71%, B1 60%, B2 19%, B3 30%, B5 27%, B6 18%,
folate 18%, biotin 15%, potassium 55%, calcium 31%, magnesium 46%, iron 68%,
zinc 33%, copper 45%, manganese 85%, selenium 2%, iodine 2%

HEALTH BENEFITS

Lowers blood cholesterol | helps maintain blood sugar levels | good for digestion

SIDE DISHES

Spiced Vegetable Parcels

Preparation and cooking time: 45 minutes | Calories per portion: 482

Serves 4

200g/7oz potatoes, cubed

1 tbsp olive oil, plus extra for greasing

1 onion, sliced

1 garlic clove, crushed

500g/1lb 2oz chestnut/cremini mushrooms, sliced

250g/9oz garden peas

1 tbsp peeled and grated root ginger

1 tsp ground coriander

1 tsp ground cumin

1 tsp garam masala

½ tsp cayenne pepper

1 tbsp amchoor or lemon juice

1 handful of fresh pomegranate seeds

375g/13oz ready-rolled puff pastry dough

1 tbsp poppy seeds

sea salt and freshly ground black pepper

Parboil the potatoes for 5 minutes, then drain. Heat the oil in a frying pan and stir-fry the onion and garlic for 1 minute. Add the mushrooms and stir-fry for a further minute, then turn the heat down and add the parboiled potatoes, the peas and all the spices except the poppy seeds. Cook gently for 5 minutes, stirring occasionally. Season.

Preheat the oven to 200°C/400°F/Gas 6. Cut the pastry dough into 4 squares and brush the edges with a little cold water. Put a spoonful of filling in the middle of each square. Fold the pastry to enclose the filling and pinch the edges together to seal. Transfer the parcels to a lightly greased baking sheet, brush with a little cold water, sprinkle with poppy seeds and bake for 20 minutes, or until puffed and golden.

NUTRIENT BALANCE (per portion)
13% protein, 43% fat, 41% carbohydrate, 3% fibre

VITAMINS AND MINERALS (percentage of RDA)
Vitamin A 14%, E 5%, C 49%, B1 51%, B2 38%, B3 41%, B5 48%, B6 49%, folate 62%, biotin 30%, potassium 50%, calcium 14%, magnesium 19%, iron 33%, zinc 20%, copper 125%, manganese 45%, selenium 24%, iodine 4%

HEALTH BENEFITS
Low in saturated fat | immune system booster | helps circulation | good for the heart and endocrine system

Roast Spiced Potato Wedges

The spices for these potato wedges are mixed together and added halfway through the cooking time to preserve their flavour.

Preparation and cooking time: 1 hour | Calories per portion: 369

Serves 4

1.5kg/3lb 5oz potatoes, scrubbed and cut
  into wedges

2 tbsp olive oil, plus extra for greasing

1 whole garlic bulb, peeled

1 tsp nigella seeds

2 tsp sweet paprika

2 tbsp balsamic vinegar

sea salt and freshly ground black pepper

Preheat the oven to 200°C/400°F/Gas 6. Put the potatoes on a lightly greased baking sheet and put in the oven to dry. Turn them after a couple of minutes and remove from the oven after 5 minutes. Sprinkle the olive oil over the potatoes, ensuring they are evenly coated. Season. Return to the oven and roast for 20 minutes.

Meanwhile, using a pestle and mortar or food processor, grind or blend the rest of the ingredients with a little oil to form a rough paste. Remove the potatoes from the oven and add the spice blend, stirring it so all the potatoes are well covered. Return to the oven for 15 minutes, or until the potatoes are crisp and golden.

Variation: Replace nigella seeds with mustard seeds for a hotter version of this dish.

NUTRIENT BALANCE (per portion)
11% protein, 17% fat, 68% carbohydrate, 4% fibre

VITAMINS AND MINERALS (percentage of RDA)
Vitamin A 26%, E 4%, C 56%, B1 76%, B2 10%, B3 18%, B6 123%, folate 66%, potassium 78%, calcium 4%, magnesium 20%, iron 20%, zinc 15%, copper 33%, selenium 8%, iodine 8%, manganese 25%

HEALTH BENEFITS
Good for chronic health problems | stimulates the immune system

Bavarian Spiced Red Cabbage

Red cabbage makes a fine accompaniment to rich roast dishes. It benefits from being stewed slowly over a long period of time

Preparation and cooking time: 1 hour | Calories per portion: 118

Serves 4

1 tbsp olive oil

1 red onion, chopped

½ red cabbage, shredded

1 red apple, cored and chopped

100ml/3½fl oz/scant ½ cup balsamic vinegar

100ml/3½fl oz/scant ½ cup elderberry cordial, undiluted

½ tsp freshly grated nutmeg

½ tsp ground cloves

½ tsp caraway seeds

sea salt and freshly ground black pepper

Heat the oil gently in a heavy pan. Add the red onion and cook gently for a few minutes to soften. Add the red cabbage and cook gently for about 5 minutes. Mix in the remaining ingredients, stirring to combine well and heat through. Bring to a gentle simmer, then cover and leave to simmer for at least 30 minutes, or longer if possible; traditionally, red cabbage is left to simmer for up to 2 hours. The cabbage should be tender and sweet.

NUTRIENT BALANCE (per portion)
7% protein, 28% fat, 52% carbohydrate, 10% fibre

VITAMINS AND MINERALS (percentage of RDA)
Vitamin C 72%, B1 6%, B3 5%, B5 5%, B6 13%, folate 22%, potassium 20%, calcium 12%, magnesium 6%, iron 11%, copper 7%, manganese 20%

HEALTH BENEFITS
Warming and comforting | rich in antioxidants | benefits the nervous system

Sweet Potato and Apple Slices

Preparation and cooking time: 50 minutes | Calories per portion: 109

Serves 4

1 tbsp olive oil, plus extra for greasing

3 sweet potatoes, peeled and sliced

2 cooking/baking apples, cored and sliced

1 tbsp grated jaggery or raw cane sugar

½ tsp ground mace

1 tsp sea salt

1 tsp melegueta peppers, crushed

Preheat the oven to 200°C/400°F/Gas 6. Lightly grease a 20 x 30cm/8 x 12in baking dish, then layer the sweet potato and apple slices in the dish. Sprinkle evenly with the jaggery, mace, salt, pepper and olive oil. Bake for 30–40 minutes, or until the potatoes and apples are tender and the top is golden.

Variations: Try pink peppercorns or 1 teaspoon of peeled and grated root ginger instead of melegueta pepper.

NUTRIENT BALANCE (per portion)
4% protein, 25% fat, 66% carbohydrate, 5% fibre

VITAMINS AND MINERALS (percentage of RDA)
Vitamin A 41%, E 3%, C 23%, B1 10%, B5 5%, B6 5%, folate 6%, potassium 13%, magnesium 5%, iron 5%, copper 14%, manganese 15%

HEALTH BENEFITS
Low in calories | energy boosting | rich in vitamin A and antioxidants | benefits digestion | stimulates circulation

Creamy Leeks and Pine Nuts

A satisfying dish that goes well with jasmine rice and seafood, fish or chicken.
It makes a good vegetarian main course with chickpeas.

Preparation and cooking time: 15 minutes | Calories per portion: 507

Serves 4

50g/1¾oz/⅓ cup pine nuts

a dash of soy sauce

1 tbsp olive oil

400ml/14fl oz/1⅔ cups coconut milk

2 tsp curry powder

500g/1lb 2oz leeks, sliced diagonally

1–2 tbsp lime juice

1 tsp green peppercorns

sea salt

coriander/cilantro leaves, to serve

Toast the pine nuts in a large dry frying pan over a medium-high heat until they start
to turn golden. Add a dash of soy sauce, then remove from the pan and leave to one
side. Heat the oil and a spoonful of the coconut milk in the same pan. Stir in the curry
powder, heat through and then add the leeks. Sauté for 2 minutes until they begin
to soften, then add the remaining coconut milk and simmer for 5 minutes, stirring
occasionally. Add the lime juice and peppercorns, season to taste. Serve sprinkled
with the toasted pine nuts and coriander/cilantro leaves.

NUTRIENT BALANCE (per portion)
8% protein, 81% fat, 9% carbohydrate, 3% fibre

VITAMINS AND MINERALS (percentage of RDA)
Vitamin A 8%, E 28%, C 53%, B1 45%, B2 9%, B3 14%, B5 3%, B6 46%, folate 37%,
biotin 4%, potassium 47%, calcium 11%, magnesium 25%, iron 46%, zinc 21%, copper 63%,
manganese 129%, selenium 4%

HEALTH BENEFITS
Energy boosting | antiviral and antibacterial | promotes wound healing | good for blood cells,
muscles and bones

Spiced Ginger Carrots

Ginger and orange add heat and sweetness to this simple carrot dish that goes well with rice, green vegetables and many main courses.

Preparation and cooking time: 20 minutes | Calories per portion: 124

Serves 4

1 tbsp olive oil

1 tsp black cumin seeds, ground

1 tsp curry powder

½ tsp sea salt

5 carrots, sliced

2.5cm/1in piece of root ginger, peeled and finely chopped

100ml/3½fl oz/scant ½ cup orange juice

1 handful of salted peanuts

freshly ground black pepper

Heat the oil in a small saucepan and add the ground black cumin, curry powder and salt. Leave to sizzle for 30 seconds, then add the carrots and ginger. Stir-fry for 1–2 minutes until the carrots are completely coated in spices, then pour in the orange juice. Cover and leave to simmer for 5–10 minutes, or until the carrots are just cooked through. Stir in the peanuts, adjust the seasoning to taste and serve immediately.

NUTRIENT BALANCE (per portion)
10% protein, 54% fat, 30% carbohydrate, 5% fibre

VITAMINS AND MINERALS (percentage of RDA)
Vitamin A 167%, E 5%, C 18%, B1 10%, B3 9%, B5 6%, B6 12%, folate 8%, biotin 17%, potassium 14%, calcium 6%, magnesium 9%, iron 17%, zinc 4%, copper 10%, manganese 18%

HEALTH BENEFITS
Benefits vision | helps improve circulation | stimulates digestion

Curried Mushrooms

An excellent side dish to accompany an Indian-inspired meal, curried mushrooms are also good as part of a spicy cooked breakfast. Quick and easy to make, they can be enjoyed on toast as a snack or with a salad for a quick lunch.

Preparation and cooking time: 15 minutes | Calories per portion: 103

Serves 4

¼ tsp asafoetida

2 tsp ground cumin

½ tsp cayenne pepper

2 tsp ground turmeric

2 tsp dried thyme

2 tbsp olive oil

500g/1lb 2oz mushrooms, quartered or halved

sea salt

Toast the spices and thyme in a large, dry frying pan over a low heat for 30 seconds, so they release their aroma. Add the oil, turn up the heat, then tip in the mushrooms and stir to cover them in the spices. Continue to cook, stirring occasionally, until the mushrooms release their moisture and start to turn golden. Season with salt to taste and serve.

NUTRIENT BALANCE (per portion)
23% protein, 61% fat, 11% carbohydrate, 6% fibre

VITAMINS AND MINERALS (percentage of RDA)
Vitamin A 9%, E 4%, B1 12%, B2 30%, B3 27%, B5 42%, B6 28%, folate 28%, biotin 30%, potassium 26%, calcium 10%, magnesium 8%, iron 44%, zinc 8%, copper 97%, manganese 22%, selenium 21%

HEALTH BENEFITS
High in protein, B vitamins and minerals | stimulates immunity | benefits skin, hair, glands, nerves and bone marrow

Japanese Asparagus

Kinpira means 'stir-fry and simmer' in Japanese and it is a method of cooking that effectively brings out the delicate flavour of asparagus.

Preparation and cooking time: 15 minutes | Calories per serving: 85

Serves 4

2 tbsp soy sauce

1 tbsp sugar

1 tbsp mirin or rice vinegar

½ tsp sansho

1 tbsp toasted sesame oil

1 large bunch of asparagus, tough ends trimmed

Mix together the soy sauce, sugar, mirin, sansho and 1 tablespoon water in a non-reactive bowl. Leave to one side.

Heat the sesame oil in a large frying pan. Add the asparagus and stir-fry over a high heat for 1 minute. Tip the soy and spice mixture into the pan, turn the heat down to low, cover and leave to simmer very gently until almost all the liquid has been absorbed and the asparagus is just beginning to soften, about 5 minutes. Serve hot.

Variations: You can substitute dry sherry for the mirin and ½ tsp ground white pepper instead of sansho. You can also add a sprinkling of lemon zest and ½ tsp chilli powder or finely chopped chilli for extra heat.

NUTRIENT BALANCE (per portion)
19% protein, 35% fat, 35% carbohydrate, 7% fibre

VITAMINS AND MINERALS (percentage of RDA)
Vitamin A 8%, E 12%, C 19%, B1 19%, B2 6%, B3 10%, B5 4%, B6 8%, folate 110%, potassium 18%, calcium 5%, magnesium 6%, iron 9%, zinc 9%, copper 12%, manganese 16%

HEALTH BENEFITS
Diuretic | anti-inflammatory | may inhibit cancer cell growth | helps prevent anaemia

Cucumber Raita

Raita is a refreshing, cooling dish designed to accompany hot, spicy meals. It also makes a tasty dip to serve with raw vegetable sticks.

Preparation and cooking time: 10 minutes | Calories per portion: 64

Serves 4

250ml/9fl oz/1 cup plain soy yogurt

½ tsp cumin seeds

1 green chilli, deseeded and finely chopped

2 tbsp chopped coriander/cilantro leaves

½ cucumber, finely sliced

sea salt

Toast the cumin seeds in a dry frying pan over a low heat, shaking the pan to ensure they don't burn, until they start to brown and release their aroma. Remove from the heat and leave to cool, then grind using a pestle and mortar or grinder. Beat the yogurt until smooth, then stir in the ground spice and remaining ingredients. Season with salt and serve chilled.

Variations: Substitute mint leaves for the coriander/cilantro and black cumin for the cumin.

NUTRIENT BALANCE (per portion)

29% protein, 43% fat, 24% carbohydrate, 3% fibre

VITAMINS AND MINERALS (percentage of RDA)

Vitamin A 4%, E 8%, C 21%, B1 4%, folate 5%, potassium 8%, calcium 4%, iron 8%, manganese 5%

HEALTH BENEFITS

Low in calories | cooling and cleansing

Pickled Ginger

Called *gari* in Japan, pickled ginger is served with sushi to cleanse the palate and enhance flavour. For best results, use firm ginger roots and slice paper-thin with a mandoline or vegetable peeler.

Preparation and cooking time: 20 minutes, plus standing | Calories per portion: 53

Serves 4

200g/7oz root ginger, peeled and sliced paper-thin
½ tsp coarse sea salt
3 tbsp rice vinegar or white wine vinegar
2 tbsp raw cane sugar

Put the finely sliced ginger in a small bowl. Sprinkle with salt and leave to stand for 30 minutes. Heat the vinegar and sugar together in a small saucepan and bring to the boil, stirring until the sugar has dissolved. Drain the ginger slices and put into a heatproof dish or sterilized jar. Pour over the hot vinegar to cover and leave to cool before serving. Alternatively, cover or seal and store in the refrigerator for up to 1 week.

NUTRIENT BALANCE (per portion)
7% protein, 6% fat, 84% carbohydrate, 3% fibre

VITAMINS AND MINERALS (percentage of RDA)
Vitamin C 3%, B3 3%, B6 6%, potassium 9%, magnesium 5%, iron 3%, copper 4%

HEALTH BENEFITS
Improves peripheral circulation | good for joints and digestion

Pickled Juniper Kiwis

An excellent preserve to serve with savoury dishes and cheese, this also makes a refreshing dessert served with pancakes, cream or ice cream.

Preparation and cooking time: 15 minutes | Calories per portion: 228

Serves 4

500g/1lb 2oz/2½ cups raw cane sugar

1 tsp juniper berries

1 lemon, peeled, pith removed, and sliced

500g/1lb 2oz kiwifruit, peeled and sliced

2.5cm/1in piece of galangal root, peeled and chopped

Put the sugar in a saucepan with the juniper berries and sliced lemon over a medium heat. Bring to the boil, then add the kiwis and galangal slices, turn the heat down to low and leave to simmer gently for 2–4 minutes. Leave to cool before serving. Alternatively, store in a sterilized jar in the refrigerator for up to 1 month.

Variation: Use root ginger instead of galangal root.

NUTRIENT BALANCE (per portion)
1% protein, 1% fat, 96% carbohydrate, 2% fibre

VITAMINS AND MINERALS (percentage of RDA)
Vitamin E 6%, C 63%, B1 2%, B5 2%, B6 3%, folate 7%, potassium 12%, calcium 6%, magnesium 5%, iron 8%, copper 10%, manganese 3%

HEALTH BENEFITS
Good for cell membranes | antibiotic | anti-inflammatory | stimulates immunity

Zedoary Pickle

Also known as *amb halad ka achar*, this spicy pickle makes an excellent accompaniment to rice dishes and Indian curries.

Preparation time: 10 minutes | Calories per portion: 6

Serves 4

4 tsp fresh zedoary root, chopped

2.5cm/1in piece of root ginger, peeled and chopped

1 small green chilli, chopped

juice of 1 lime

½ tsp sea salt

Put all the ingredients in a pestle and mortar or food processor, and grind or whizz to a coarse paste. Serve immediately or cover and store in the refrigerator for a few days.

Variation: Try using fresh turmeric or galangal root instead of zedoary.

NUTRIENT BALANCE (per portion)
21% protein, 15% fat, 60% carbohydrate, 4% fibre

VITAMINS AND MINERALS (percentage of RDA)
Vitamin C 11%

HEALTH BENEFITS
Antioxidant | anti-inflammatory | stimulates circulation | promotes sweating

Fresh Curry Leaf Chutney

Preparation and cooking time: 20 minutes | Calories per portion: 135

Serves 8

3 tbsp split red lentils

50g/1½oz/1 packed cup fresh curry leaves

1 tsp tamarind paste

100g/3½oz fresh coconut flesh, chopped

1 small green chilli

1 tsp coconut oil

1 tsp mustard seeds

a pinch of asafoetida

sea salt

Toast the lentils and curry leaves in a dry, heavy pan over a low heat for 1–2 minutes, shaking the pan to ensure they don't burn, until the lentils darken and the leaves curl and go crisp. Mix in the tamarind, then remove from the heat and leave to cool. Grind to a fine paste with the coconut, green chilli, salt and a little water.

Heat the coconut oil with the mustard seeds and asafoetida until the mustard seeds pop, then mix into the curry paste. Serve immediately or cover and store in the refrigerator for a few days.

Serve with Indian bread or pancakes, as a snack or as a side dish.

Variations: Use split white lentils or split yellow peas instead of red lentils. Remove the chilli seeds for a milder version.

NUTRIENT BALANCE (per portion)
12% protein, 62% fat, 22% carbohydrate, 4% fibre

VITAMINS AND MINERALS (percentage of RDA)
Vitamin A 18%, C 6%, B1 6%, B2 4%, B3 4%, B5 3%, B6 4%, folate 11%, potassium 8%, calcium 15%, magnesium 12%, iron 15%, zinc 5%, copper 18%, manganese 19%, selenium 5%

HEALTH BENEFITS
Antioxidant | good for eyes, blood and bones | stimulates circulation | promotes healthy digestion

Mango and Coconut Salsa

Preparation time: 10 minutes, plus chilling | Calories per portion: 197

Serves 4

1 mango, peeled, pitted and chopped

½ tsp grated jaggery or muscovado/brown sugar

zest and juice of 1 lime

200g/7oz fresh coconut flesh, shaved

2 red chillies, deseeded and finely sliced

1 handful of coriander/cilantro leaves, chopped

Gently mix together all the ingredients in a non-reactive bowl, cover and refrigerate for 15–30 minutes to let the flavours develop.

Serve with savoury rice dishes.

NUTRIENT BALANCE (per portion)
5% protein, 52% fat, 37% carbohydrate, 5% fibre

VITAMINS AND MINERALS (percentage of RDA)
Vitamin A 20%, E 10%, C 74%, B1 7%, B2 6%, B3 6%, B5 5%, B6 14%, folate 6%, potassium 21%, calcium 4%, magnesium 8%, iron 13%, zinc 5%, copper 30%, manganese 42%, selenium 6%

HEALTH BENEFITS
Strongly antioxidant and antibiotic | immune system booster | anti-inflammatory

DESSERTS AND BAKING

Mahlepi Syrup

A Greek recipe, mahlepi syrup goes well with yogurt, ice cream, fruit salad and pancakes.

Preparation and cooking time: 20 minutes | Calories per portion: 121

Serves 4

4 tbsp grated jaggery or muscovado/brown sugar

4 tbsp honey

4 tbsp lemon juice

1 tbsp mahlepi, freshly ground

Put all the ingredients in a small saucepan with 60ml/2fl oz/¼ cup water and bring to the boil. Turn the heat down to low and leave to simmer until the syrup has thickened. Strain and cool before serving.

Variations: If you can't find mahlepi, try substituting with ground almonds, ground cardamom or fennel seeds.

NUTRIENT BALANCE (per portion)

3% protein, 11% fat, 85% carbohydrate, 1% fibre

VITAMINS AND MINERALS (percentage of RDA)

Vitamin E 5%, C 7%, B2 3%, folate 2%, biotin 4%, potassium 5%, calcium 3%, magnesium 7%, iron 3%, zinc 2%, copper 15%, manganese 8%

HEALTH BENEFITS

Digestive tonic | calms the nerves

Griddled Pineapple

A refreshing treat that is quick to cook on a griddle/grill pan or barbecue.

Preparation and cooking time: 20 minutes | Calories per portion: 173

Serves 4

100g/3½oz grated jaggery or muscovado/soft brown sugar

1 vanilla pod/bean

a pinch of saffron strands, crushed

1 ripe pineapple, sliced into long wedges, skin and core removed

Heat the jaggery and 200ml/7fl oz/scant 1 cup water in a saucepan over a medium-high heat, stirring regularly until the sugar has dissolved. Add the vanilla pod/bean and saffron. Bring to the boil, then turn the heat down to low and leave to simmer gently for 10 minutes, or until the liquid has thickened to a syrup.

Put the pineapple slices in a bowl and pour over the syrup. Leave to marinate while you heat a griddle/grill pan to hot. Put the slices in the pan and cook for 2 minutes on each side. Serve with marinade syrup drizzled over.

NUTRIENT BALANCE (per portion)
2% protein, 2% fat, 94% carbohydrate, 2% fibre

VITAMINS AND MINERALS (percentage of RDA)
Vitamin C 24%, B1 14%, B2 4%, B3 3%, B5 4%, B6 10%, folate 4%, potassium 17%, calcium 7%, magnesium 15%, iron 6%, zinc 2%, copper 37%, manganese 61%

HEALTH BENEFITS
Improves digestion | helps relieve constipation | antioxidant and mildly sedative

Wasabi Apple Crumble Surprise

In this new take on an old favourite, the wasabi brings out the flavour of the apples and enhances their sweetness.

Preparation and cooking time: 45 minutes | Calories per portion: 464

Serves 8

500g/1lb 2oz cooking/baking apples, peeled, cored and sliced

50g/1½oz jaggery, grated or 50g/1½oz/¼ cup soft dark brown sugar

1 tsp grated fresh wasabi, or ½ tsp dried

½ tsp ground cinnamon

100g/3½oz dark/bittersweet chocolate, broken into pieces

For the topping

300g/10½oz/2¼ cups plain/all-purpose flour

200g/7oz jaggery, grated, or 200g/7oz/ 1 cup muscovado/brown sugar

a pinch of fine sea salt

200g/7oz vegetable margarine, cut into cubes, plus extra for greasing

Preheat the oven to 180°C/350°F/Gas 4 and grease a large ovenproof dish. To make the topping, mix the flour, sugar and salt together in a large bowl. Add the margarine and rub it into the flour until it forms small lumps.

Prepare the apples and put the slices into the prepared dish. Add the sugar, wasabi and cinnamon and mix together well so the apple slices are coated in spices and sugar. Scatter over the chocolate pieces, then tip in the crumble topping and smooth it over in a thick layer. Bake for 30 minutes, or until the top is golden and the apple mixture is bubbling underneath.

Variations: You can use grated horseradish to replace the wasabi, and cassia instead of cinnamon.

NUTRIENT BALANCE (per portion)

4% protein, 41% fat, 53% carbohydrate, 1% fibre

VITAMINS AND MINERALS (percentage of RDA)

Vitamin A 22%, E 3%, C 11%, B1 12%, B2 2%, B3 4%, B5 2%, B6 7%, folate 6%, biotin 3%, potassium 9%, calcium 9%, magnesium 7%, iron 12%, zinc 4%, copper 17%, manganese 15%, selenium 2%

HEALTH BENEFITS

Antioxidant | stimulates circulation | good for lungs and respiration

Oriental Poached Pears

Preparation and cooking time: 45 minutes, plus cooling | Calories per portion: 308

Serves 4

100ml/3½fl oz/scant ½ cup maple syrup

4 tbsp grated jaggery or muscovado/
  brown sugar

3 tbsp lemon juice

1 tbsp white wine vinegar

4 star anise

5cm/2in piece of cassia bark

2 tbsp dried galangal root

4 nashi pears (Asian or Chinese pears),
  peeled and cored

2 mangoes, peeled, pitted and sliced

100g/3½oz/¾ cup hazelnuts,
  toasted and chopped

Put the maple syrup, jaggery, lemon juice, vinegar and spices in a saucepan with 500ml/17fl oz/2 cups water. Bring to the boil, stirring, then turn the heat down to medium-low and leave to simmer for 5 minutes, or until the jaggery dissolves. Add the pears and simmer gently for 30 minutes, or until tender. Leave to cool before serving.

Divide the mango slices among four plates. Remove the cooled pears from the syrup and put on top of the mango slices. Strain the spiced syrup over the pears and sprinkle with the toasted hazelnuts.

Variations: You can substitute any plump pears for the nashi pears, and root ginger for the galangal.

NUTRIENT BALANCE (per portion)
5% protein, 32% fat, 57% carbohydrate, 5% fibre

VITAMINS AND MINERALS (percentage of RDA)
Vitamin A 30/%, E 43%, C 90%, B1 15%, B2 12%, B3 9%, B5 9%, B6 25%, folate 7%, biotin 17%, potassium 33%, calcium 11%, magnesium 17%, iron 26%, zinc 11%, copper 52%, manganese 83%

HEALTH BENEFITS
Antioxidant | rich in micronutrients | good for eyes, skin, nails, hair and mucous membranes | stimulates circulation

Sweet Coconut Blinis

Gram flour is made from chickpeas and gives a soft, rich texture to these Indian-inspired sweet pancakes. They are good served with preserves and whipped coconut cream, or slices of fresh fruit.

Preparation and cooking time: 30 minutes | Calories per portion: 246

Serves 4

150g/5½oz/1¼ cups chickpea (gram) flour

50g/1¾oz/¾ cup desiccated/dried
   shredded coconut

1 tsp ground cinnamon

seeds from 1 vanilla pod/bean or ½ tsp
   vanilla powder

½ tsp ground allspice

a pinch of fine sea salt

3 tbsp soy milk

1 tbsp honey

1–2 tbsp coconut or corn oil

Mix the dry ingredients together in a bowl. Make a well in the middle and gradually beat in the milk, honey and 80ml/2½fl oz/⅓ cup water to form a medium-thick batter. Leave the batter to stand for 15 minutes, then mix again to a smooth consistency (adding a little more water if necessary) just before cooking.

Heat 1 tablespoon of the oil in a frying pan over a medium heat. Pour a few tablespoonfuls of batter into the hot pan to make several small, round pancakes and cook for 1–2 minutes, turning them over as they become firm and golden. Remove the blinis from the pan and keep warm wrapped in foil or in a low oven while you add a little more oil to the pan and repeat with the remaining batter. Serve hot.

NUTRIENT BALANCE (per portion)
17% protein, 39% fat, 38% carbohydrate, 6% fibre

VITAMINS AND MINERALS (percentage of RDA)
Vitamin E 5%, B1 19%, B2 6%, B3 5%, B5 5%, B6 16%, folate 89%, potassium 23%, calcium 6%, magnesium 22%, iron 22%, zinc 13%, copper 45%, manganese 49%, selenium 9%

HEALTH BENEFITS
Packed with micronutrients | good for nerves, muscles, blood cells and joints

Oranges in Spicy Wine Syrup

Preparation and cooking time: 30 minutes, plus chilling | Calories per portion: 172

Serves 4

250ml/9fl oz/1 cup red wine

50g/1¾oz jaggery, grated, or raw cane sugar

4 allspice berries

8 black peppercorns

1 cinnamon stick

4 whole cloves

4 star anise

zest of 1 orange

4 oranges, peel and pith removed and sliced into rings

Heat the wine gently in a saucepan with the sugar and spices, stirring until all the sugar has dissolved. Add the orange zest and bring to the boil, then turn the heat down to medium and leave to simmer gently for 10 minutes, or until the liquid has reduced to a syrup. Strain to remove the whole spices, then leave to cool.

Put the orange slices in a bowl, pour over the cooled syrup, cover and chill in the refrigerator for at least 2 hours, or overnight. Take out of the refrigerator 30 minutes before serving.

NUTRIENT BALANCE (per portion)

12% protein, 4% fat, 79% carbohydrate, 5% fibre

VITAMINS AND MINERALS (percentage of RDA)

Vitamin C 81%, B1 13%, B2 5%, B3 4%, B5 8%, B6 10%, folate 19%, biotin 5%, potassium 19%, calcium 16%, magnesium 12%, iron 15%, zinc 4%, copper 25%, manganese 24%, selenium 3%, iodine 2%

HEALTH BENEFITS

Antioxidant | improves digestion | enhances resistance to infection

Chocolate and Avocado Mousse

Preparation time: 10 minutes | Calories per portion: 183

Serves 4

2 avocados, peeled, pitted and sliced

2 tbsp unsweetened cocoa powder

seeds from 1 vanilla pod/bean or 1 tsp vanilla powder

2 tbsp maple syrup

4 tbsp almond milk

1 handful of mint leaves

fresh pomegranate seeds

Put all the ingredients, except the pomegranate seeds, in a blender or food processor and blend together to form a smooth, light mousse. Divide the mousse among four sundae glasses, sprinkle over the pomegranate seeds and serve. Alternatively, cover and refrigerate until needed.

NUTRIENT BALANCE (per portion)
8% protein, 63% fat, 19% carbohydrate, 9% fibre

VITAMINS AND MINERALS (percentage of RDA)
Vitamin A 6%, E 25%, C 17%, B1 8%, B2 11%, B3 10%, B5 18%, B6 16%, folate 40%, potassium 27%, calcium 9%, magnesium 16%, iron 20%, zinc 13%, copper 44%, manganese 28%

HEALTH BENEFITS
Excellent source of beneficial fats | helps maintain blood sugar level | antioxidant | protects heart and circulation | may help lower blood cholesterol

Tamarind Ice Cream

This recipe requires an ice cream maker for best results.

Preparation and cooking time: 30 minutes, plus cooling and freezing | Calories per portion: 267

Serves 4

250g/9oz jaggery, finely grated, or muscovado/brown sugar
3 egg yolks
650ml/22fl oz/2¾ cups coconut cream
100ml/3½fl oz/scant ½ cup tamarind paste

Using an electric hand whisk/beater, beat the jaggery and egg yolks together in a bowl until the mixture is pale and smooth.

Pour the coconut cream into a saucepan, add the tamarind paste and heat over a medium heat to a gentle simmer; do not let it boil. Remove from the heat, add the sugar mixture and beat until well combined. Return to a low heat and cook for 8–10 minutes, or until the mixture has thickened enough to coat the back of a spoon. Leave to cool completely.

Pour the cooled mixture into the bowl of your ice cream maker and freeze according to the manufacturer's instructions. Remove the ice cream from the freezer about 20 minutes before serving.

NUTRIENT BALANCE (per portion)
4% protein, 54% fat, 41% carbohydrate, 1% fibre

VITAMINS AND MINERALS (percentage of RDA)
Vitamin A 2%, D 3%, E 3%, C 2%, B1 4%, B2 3%, B3 3%, B5 2%, folate 2%, biotin 3%, potassium 11%, calcium 5%, magnesium 12%, iron 13%, zinc 6%, copper 33%, manganese 33%, selenium 2%, iodine 3%

HEALTH BENEFITS
Rich in beneficial plant oils | good for digestion and respiration

Quick Banana Muffins

Preparation and cooking time: 35 minutes | Calories per portion: 285

Makes 20 mini muffins

125g/4½oz vegetable margarine, melted

150g/5½oz/¾ cup raw cane sugar

1 tsp vanilla seeds, scraped from a pod/bean

3 bananas, cut into small chunks

1 egg, lightly beaten (optional)

100ml/3½fl oz/scant ½ cup soy, almond or rice milk

200g/7oz/1½ cups plain/all-purpose flour

2 tsp baking powder

½ tsp fine sea salt

Preheat the oven to 200°C/400°F/Gas 6 and set out 20 small paper cake cases/ liners on a baking sheet. In a bowl, combine the margarine, sugar, vanilla, bananas, egg and milk. Don't worry about any lumps of banana – they will enhance the taste and texture of the muffins. Sift together the flour and baking powder in a separate bowl and make a well in the middle. Pour the wet ingredients into the flour and mix until just combined. Spoon in the batter to half fill each muffin case/liner. Bake for about 20 minutes until risen and golden. Transfer to a wire/cooling rack to cool slightly before serving.

NUTRIENT BALANCE (per portion)
6% protein, 40% fat, 52% carbohydrate, 2% fibre

VITAMINS AND MINERALS (percentage of RDA)
Vitamin A 15%, D 24%, E 3%, C 5%, B1 10%, B2 6%, B3 7%, B5 5%, folate 10%, biotin 5%, potassium 12%, calcium 7%, magnesium 9%, iron 9%, zinc 6%, copper 13%, manganese 28%, selenium 3%, iodine 4%

HEALTH BENEFITS
Nutrient rich | promotes steady energy release

Spiced Sister Cake

In the old farmhouse where I live, there once lived a widow called Maren.
She baked the most delicious spice cake, and this is her recipe. I use fresh yeast
but if you have fast-action/instant active dried yeast, just follow the instructions
on the package.

Preparation and cooking time: 50 minutes, plus rising | Calories per portion: 364

Serves 8

100ml/3½fl oz/scant 1 cup milk

25g/1oz fresh yeast

150g/5½oz vegetable margarine, plus extra
  for greasing

25g/1oz raw cane sugar

1 egg, lightly beaten

50g/1¾oz/⅓ cup raisins

25g/1oz candied peel

½ tsp ground cardamom

½ tsp ground cloves

½ tsp ground allspice

1 tsp peeled and grated root ginger

250g/9oz/scant 2 cups plain/all-
  purpose flour

To decorate

1 apple, cored and cubed

3 tbsp raw cane sugar

1 tsp ground cinnamon

1 handful of flaked/sliced almonds, chopped

Heat the milk gently until hand-hot, then pour into a large bowl. Add the yeast and
leave it to foam and dissolve, then mix in all the remaining ingredients and knead to
a soft dough. Shape into a ball, cover and leave to rise in a warm place for about
40 minutes, or until double in size.

Preheat the oven to 200°C/400°F/Gas 6. Grease a round 23cm/9in cake pan.
Transfer the risen dough to the greased pan and pat it down so it covers the bottom
up to the edges. Make several cuts in the dough to let it rise evenly and avoid cracks.

Roll the apple cubes in the sugar and cinnamon and sprinkle over the top of the cake
with the chopped almonds. Bake in the middle of the oven for about 30 minutes, or
until golden and baked through.

NUTRIENT BALANCE (per portion)

9% protein, 49% fat, 39% carbohydrate, 3% fibre

VITAMINS AND MINERALS (percentage of RDA)

Vitamin A 19%, D 30%, E 16%, C 1%, B1 17%, B2 14%, B3 12%, B5 7%, folate 32%, biotin 17%, potassium 14%, calcium 11%, magnesium 15%, iron 19%, zinc 11%, copper 28%, manganese 44%, selenium 5%, iodine 3%

HEALTH BENEFITS

Nutrient rich I improves general immunity I good for hair, nails, blood and bones

Welsh Cakes

These delicious cakes are a traditional Welsh teatime treat. Packed with cinnamon, nutmeg and dried fruit, they are best served warm.

Preparation and cooking time: 25 minutes | Calories per portion: 316

Serves 4

250g/9oz/scant 2 cups plain/all-purpose flour, plus extra for dusting

1 tsp baking powder

50g/1¾oz vegetable margarine, cut into cubes, plus extra for greasing

50g/1¾oz solid coconut oil, cut into cubes

100g/3½oz grated jaggery or 100g/3½oz/½ cup muscovado/brown sugar

1 handful of raisins

1 tsp ground cinnamon

1 tsp ground nutmeg

1 egg, beaten

oil, for frying

icing/confectioners' sugar for dusting

Sift the flour and baking powder together into a large mixing bowl. Rub in the margarine and coconut oil with your fingertips until the mixture resembles fine breadcrumbs. Mix in the jaggery, raisins, cinnamon and nutmeg. Add the beaten egg or 50ml/1¾fl oz/scant ¼ cup water and mix into a smooth ball of dough, adding a little more water if the texture is too dry.

Put the dough on a lightly floured surface and knead until smooth, then roll it out until 5mm/¼in thick. Using an 8cm/3in cutter or upturned cup, cut out rounds. Re-roll the trimmings to cut out more.

Heat a little oil in a large heavy frying pan. When hot, add as many cakes as you can fit with space between them. Cook for about 3 minutes on each side until crisp, golden and cooked through. Repeat with the remaining cakes. Dust with icing/confectioners' sugar and serve warm.

Variations: You can replace the nutmeg with mace, and the cinnamon with cassia. For a vegan version, you can use a natural egg replacer, such as No Egg.

NUTRIENT BALANCE (per portion)

6% protein, 36% fat, 57% carbohydrate, 1% fibre

VITAMINS AND MINERALS (percentage of RDA)

Vitamin A 7%, D 12%, B1 11%, B2 3%, B3 3%, B5 3%, folate 5%, biotin 3%, potassium 11%, calcium 11%, magnesium 8%, iron 12%, zinc 4%, copper 21%, manganese 18%, selenium 4%, iodine 4%

HEALTH BENEFITS

Helps maintain steady energy | good for bones

Saffron Buns

Saffron buns are popular throughout Scandinavia, where they are baked in an 'S' shape and known as Santa Lucia buns or *Lussekatter* because they are served at the Santa Lucia celebration of light. If you have fast-action/instant active dried yeast, just follow the instructions on the package.

Preparation and baking time: 40 minutes, plus rising | Calories per portion: 220

Makes 14

300ml/10½fl oz/1¼ cups almond milk

65g/2¼oz vegetable margarine

a large pinch of saffron strands

25g/1oz fresh yeast

100ml/3½fl oz/scant ½ cup plain yogurt

100g/3½oz/½ cup raw cane sugar

1 tsp ground cinnamon

a pinch of freshly grated nutmeg

½ tsp fine sea salt

200g/7oz/1½ cups dried currants, plus extra to decorate

500g/1lb 2oz/3¾ cups plain/all-purpose flour

1 egg, beaten, or 1 tbsp cold coffee

Warm the milk and margarine in a saucepan over a medium heat. Stir in the saffron, then take off the heat and leave to infuse and cool a little. When lukewarm, pour the milk mixture into a large bowl and add the yeast. When the yeast has dissolved, stir in the yogurt, sugar, spices, salt and currants. Mix in the flour a little at a time to form a dough, then knead to a light, elastic consistency. Shape into a ball, then cover with cling film/plastic wrap and leave to rise in a warm place for about 40 minutes, or until double in size.

Line a baking sheet with baking parchment. Divide the dough into 14 pieces and roll each one to form a 10cm/4in sausage. Curl each end in opposite directions to make an 'S' shape. Transfer to the prepared baking sheet, cover with cling film/plastic wrap and leave to rise for 30 minutes.

Preheat the oven to 225°C/425°F/Gas 7. Brush the buns with the egg, decorate with a currant in the curl at each end, then bake for about 8 minutes, or until golden. Leave to cool for a few minutes, then serve warm, split and buttered, if you like.

Variation: For a vegan version, you can use a natural egg replacer, such as No Egg.

NUTRIENT BALANCE (per portion)
8% protein, 18% fat, 72% carbohydrate, 2% fibre

VITAMINS AND MINERALS (percentage of RDA)
Vitamin A 7%, D 6%, E 9%, B1 12%, B2 3%, B3 5%, B5 3%, folate 14%, biotin 4%, potassium 9%, calcium 11%, magnesium 4%, iron 9%, zinc 3%, copper 19%, manganese 20%, selenium 1%, iodine 2%

HEALTH BENEFITS
May help lower blood cholesterol | warming and soothing

Armenian Brioche

These Armenian rolls are best served hot. I use fresh yeast in the recipe, but if you have fast-action/instant active dried yeast, just follow the instructions on the package.

Preparation and cooking time: 40 minutes, plus rising | Calories per portion: 233

Makes 12

25g/1oz fresh yeast	1 egg, lightly beaten, plus extra for brushing
1 tbsp sugar	1 tbsp ground mahlab
a pinch of fine sea salt	100g/3½oz vegetable margarine, cut
2 tbsp almond milk	into cubes
250g/9oz/scant 2 cups spelt flour	2 tbsp poppy seeds

For the filling

100g/3½oz/¾ cup pitted dates, chopped	a pinch of ground cloves
50g/1¾oz/⅓ cup walnuts, chopped	1 tbsp honey
½ tsp ground cassia	

Crumble the yeast into a cup and stir in 2 tablespoons warm water. Leave to stand for 10 minutes until the yeast has dissolved. In a separate bowl, stir the sugar and salt into the cold milk. Sift in the flour, make a well in the middle and add the beaten egg followed by the yeast mixture. Gently mix everything together, then add the mahlab spice and the margarine, a third at a time, until you have a smooth and elastic dough. Adjust the consistency with more milk or flour, if necessary. Shape into a ball, then cover with cling film/plastic wrap and leave to rise in a warm place for about 40 minutes, or until double in size.

Knead the risen dough lightly, then leave for a further 10 minutes to rise again. Meanwhile, mix together all the filling ingredients in a bowl.

Line a baking sheet with baking parchment. Divide the dough into 12 balls. Flatten each one between the palms of your hands. Put a spoonful of the filling in the middle of each ball and pull the edges up and over the filling. Pinch the edges together to seal the balls, then transfer to the prepared baking sheet. Leave to rest for 20 minutes.

Preheat the oven to 200°C/400°F/Gas 6. Brush the rolls with beaten egg, sprinkle with the poppy seeds and bake for 15–20 minutes, or until the rolls are firm and golden.

Tip: If you can't find mahlab, use ground almonds instead.

Variation: For a vegan version, you can use a natural egg replacer, such as No Egg.

NUTRIENT BALANCE (per portion)
9% protein, 48% fat, 39% carbohydrate, 4% fibre

VITAMINS AND MINERALS (percentage of RDA)
Vitamin A 10%, D 15%, E 7%, B1 11%, B2 7%, B3 8%, B5 6%, folate 20%, biotin 9%, potassium 10%, calcium 10%, magnesium 11%, iron 12%, zinc 10%, copper 25%, manganese 41%, selenium 3%, iodine 2%

HEALTH BENEFITS
Rich in health-promoting oils, vitamins and minerals | improves wellbeing | helps calm nerves and digestion | strongly antioxidant

Tuscan Panforte

Preparation and cooking time: 50 minutes | Calories per portion: 332

Serves 8

50g/1¾oz/heaped ⅓ cup spelt flour

½ tsp ground cinnamon

1 tsp ground aniseed

½ tsp vanilla seeds, scraped from a pod/bean

a pinch of cayenne pepper

200g/7oz/1¾ cups dried figs, chopped

50g/1¾oz/⅓ cup almonds

50g/1¾oz/⅓ cup hazelnuts, chopped

50g/1¾oz/⅓ cup walnuts, chopped

100g/3½ oz dark/bittersweet chocolate, chopped

1 tsp orange zest

5 tbsp syrup or honey

3 tbsp raw cane sugar or grated jaggery

2 tbsp orange juice

cocoa powder and icing sugar, for dusting

Preheat the oven to 150°C/300°F/Gas 2. Grease a 15cm/6in cake pan and line it with baking parchment. Sift the flour and spices into a mixing bowl. Add the figs, nuts, chocolate and orange zest and mix in gently. In a small saucepan, heat the honey, sugar and orange juice and simmer for about 5 minutes, stirring continuously, until the sugar dissolves. Pour the melted honey mixture over the dry ingredients and mix together quickly. Spoon into the prepared tin and bake for 35–40 minutes, or until the edges are firm and raised higher than the middle.

Leave to cool completely in the pan, then turn it out, peel off the paper and dust with cocoa and icing sugar before serving.

NUTRIENT BALANCE (per portion)
4% protein, 54% fat, 41% carbohydrate, 1% fibre

VITAMINS AND MINERALS (percentage of RDA)
Vitamin A 4%, E 29%, C 3%, B1 10%, B2 8%, B3 5%, B5 7%, folate 9%, biotin 21%, potassium 23%, calcium 15%, magnesium 19%, iron 20%, zinc 10%, copper 41%, manganese 47%, selenium 2%, iodine 2%

HEALTH BENEFITS
Rich in micronutrients and unsaturated fats | warming and soothing

Fennel Fougasse

A traditional Provençal bread similar to Italian focaccia.

Preparation and cooking time: 50 minutes, plus rising | Calories per portion: 256

Serves 8

25g/1oz fresh yeast

1 tsp sea salt

1 tsp syrup or honey

500g/1lb 2oz/3¾ cups spelt flour

1 tbsp fennel seeds, lightly toasted and
crushed

2 tbsp olive oil, plus extra for greasing

1 tbsp nigella seeds or poppy seeds

Put the yeast and 200ml/7fl oz/scant 1cup tepid water in a large bowl and leave to stand for a few minutes, until it has dissolved. Stir in the salt and honey, followed by the flour, fennel seeds and 1 tablespoon of the oil. Knead to form a soft dough, then cover with a clean dish towel and leave to rise in a warm place for at least 1 hour.

Preheat the oven to 220°C/425°F/Gas 7 and grease a baking sheet. Turn out the dough onto a floured surface. Dust with a little more flour, roll out to a flat rectangle and put on the prepared baking sheet. Leave to rise for 10 minutes, then brush with the remaining oil and sprinkle over the nigella seeds. Bake for 10 minutes, then remove from the oven, partially baked, and cover with a damp dish towel for a few minutes. Cut several long slits in the bread, about 3cm/1¼in apart and 3cm/1¼in from the edges. Return the bread to the oven and bake for 10–15 minutes, or until the surface is crisp and golden. Cool on a wire/cooling rack before serving.

NUTRIENT BALANCE (per portion)
15% protein, fat 18%, carbohydrate 62%, 5% fibre

VITAMINS AND MINERALS (percentage of RDA)
Vitamin E 5%, B1 26%, B2 8%, B3 19%, B5 6%, B6 15%, folate 35%, biotin 7%, potassium 11%, calcium 17%, magnesium 18%, iron 19%, zinc 15%, copper 30%, manganese 72%, selenium 5%

HEALTH BENEFITS
Good for bones, skin, hair and nails | calms digestion

DRINKS

Spiced Tisane

Preparation time: 10 minutes | Calories per serving: 36

Serves 4

2.5cm/1in piece of root ginger, peeled and chopped or grated

3 cardamom pods, crushed

1 cinnamon stick

1 lemongrass stalk

5 whole cloves

Put the spices in a teapot or saucepan. Add 1l/35fl oz/4¼ cups boiling water and leave to infuse for at least 7 minutes. Pour into cups, using a tea strainer or small sieve/fine-mesh strainer to catch the spices. Serve hot.

NUTRIENT BALANCE (per portion)
10% protein, 22% fat, 45% carbohydrate, 23% fibre

VITAMINS AND MINERALS (percentage of RDA)
Vitamin B1 2%, B2 2%, B3 2%, B5 2%, B6 2%, folate 2%, potassium 8%, calcium 11%, magnesium 6%, iron 34%, copper 9%, manganese 46%

HEALTH BENEFITS
Warming and stimulating for circulation and digestion | strongly antioxidant | immune system booster | helps to prevent colds and flu

Fennel Tisane

A fennel tisane is warming and aids digestion.

Preparation time: 10 minutes | Calories per serving: 19

Serves 1

1 tsp fennel seeds, lightly crushed

1 slice of lemon, to serve

Put the fennel seeds in a tea filter in a mug or small teapot. Add 250 ml/9fl oz/ 1 cup boiling water and leave to infuse for 5 minutes. Serve hot with a slice of lemon.

NUTRIENT BALANCE (per portion)

19% protein, 37% fat, 19% carbohydrate, 25% fibre

VITAMINS AND MINERALS (percentage of RDA)

Vitamin C 9%, B1 2%, B3 3%, potassium 5%, calcium 8%, magnesium 6%, iron 5%, copper 5%, manganese 16%

HEALTH BENEFITS

Helps digestion, relieving wind and colic | aids slimming

Star Anise Tisane

This sweet and refreshing tisane is a natural immunity booster and digestive aid. Delicious all year round, it is best made with fresh ingredients at the beginning of summer, when the elder blooms.

Preparation and cooking time: 10 minutes | Calories per serving: 32

Serves 4

4 star anise

1 cluster of fresh elderflowers, rinsed, or 1 tsp dried

1cm/½in piece of root ginger, peeled and grated

1 cinnamon stick

3 peppermint sprigs, or 1 tsp dried

1 tbsp orange zest

Put all the ingredients in a tea bag or tea filter, then set in a large teapot. Bring 1l/35fl oz/4¼ cups water to the boil, leave to stand for 1 minute, then pour over the spices. Cover and leave to infuse for 5 minutes before pouring.

Variation: To make a cocktail with this infusion, cool and served on ice with a splash of single malt whisky and some soda.

NUTRIENT BALANCE (per portion)
14% protein, 17% fat, 49% carbohydrate, 20% fibre

VITAMINS AND MINERALS (percentage of RDA)
Vitamin C 23%, B1 2%, B2 3%, B3 2%, B5 2%, B6 3%, folate 8%, potassium 7%, calcium 10%, magnesium 4%, iron 16%, zinc 3%, copper 7%, manganese 13%

HEALTH BENEFITS
A good flu remedy | stimulates circulation | helps to reduce fever

Black Cumin Coffee

In the Middle East, coffee is often served with a pinch of black cumin to add a spicy, peppery note. The cumin can be ground with the coffee beans or simply added to the filter or cafetière.

Preparation time: 4 minutes | Calories per serving: 10

Serves 1

1 tbsp coffee beans, ground
½ tsp black cumin seeds, ground

Mix the coffee beans and the cumin seeds together and put in a cafetière or coffee filter. Pour in 250ml/9fl oz/1 cup boiling water and leave to stand for 5 minutes, then filter and serve.

NUTRIENT BALANCE (per portion)
28% protein, 46% fat, 34% carbohydrate, 5% fibre

VITAMINS AND MINERALS (percentage of RDA)
Vitamin B1 5%, B2 14%, B3 4%, B5 11%, folate 3%, potassium 8%, calcium 4%, magnesium 4%, iron 13%, copper 4%, manganese 7%

HEALTH BENEFITS
Effective digestive and liver stimulant | helps improve fat digestion

Solkadhi

A refreshing, soothing and cooling drink that is popular in India.

Preparation and cooking time: 15 minutes, plus cooling | Calories per serving: 258

Serves 4

5 kokum slices
400ml/14fl oz/1⅔ cups coconut milk
100ml/3½fl oz/scant ½ cup plain soy yogurt
2 green chillies, crushed
1 garlic clove, crushed
¼ tsp ground cumin
sugar, to taste
sea salt

Bring 200ml/7fl oz/scant 1 cup water to the boil in a small saucepan. Add the kokum slices, turn the heat down and to simmer for 5 minutes. Strain, reserving the liquid, and leave to cool.

Meanwhile, put all the remaining ingredients in a blender and blend together until smooth. Add the cooled kokum liquid and adjust the seasoning to taste. Serve immediately or chill before serving.

NUTRIENT BALANCE (per portion)
7% protein, 79% fat, 13% carbohydrate, 1% fibre

VITAMINS AND MINERALS (percentage of RDA)
Vitamin A 2%, E 4%, C 9%, B1 4%, B2 2%, B3 6%, B5 3%, B6 4%, folate 8%, potassium 17%, calcium 4%, magnesium 15%, iron 30%, zinc 7%, copper 27%, manganese 42%

HEALTH BENEFITS
Rich and nourishing | helps reduce inflammation | antioxidant and antiviral

Strawberry Lassi

Preparation time: 5 minutes | Calories per serving: 289

Serves 4

400ml/14fl oz/1⅔ cups plain soy yogurt

200g/7oz strawberries, hulled

50g/1½oz grated jaggery or raw cane sugar

½ tsp vanilla seeds, scraped from a pod/bean

Put the yogurt, strawberries, jaggery and vanilla seeds in a blender and blend until smooth. Thin with a little water, if you like, and serve with ice cubes or a few frozen strawberries.

NUTRIENT BALANCE (per portion)

18% protein, 28% fat, 52% carbohydrate, 2% fibre

VITAMINS AND MINERALS (percentage of RDA)

Vitamin A 6%, E 28%, C 96%, B1 4%, B2 8%, B3 4%, B5 6%, B6 6%, folate 12%, potassium 13%, calcium 5%, magnesium 12%, iron 6%, zinc 2%, copper 27%, manganese 23%, iodine 6%

HEALTH BENEFITS

Antioxidant | immune system booster | may help to inhibit cancer cell growth

Zedoary Juice

Zedoary root has a delicate and distinct flavour and makes a great immune-boosting energy drink, mixed with maple syrup and lime.

Preparation time: 5 minutes, plus chilling | Calories per serving: 295

Serves 4

5cm/2in piece of zedoary root, peeled and chopped

1 tbsp maple syrup

1 banana

juice from 1 lime

5 kaffir lime leaves

a pinch of sea salt

500ml/17fl oz/2 cups coconut juice

Put all the ingredients in a blender and blend until smooth. Serve chilled.

NUTRIENT BALANCE (per portion)
5% protein, 82% fat, 13% carbohydrate, 1% fibre

VITAMINS AND MINERALS (percentage of RDA)
Vitamin C 12%, B1 4%, B3 7%, B5 5%, B6 8%, folate 11%, potassium 24%, calcium 4%, magnesium 20%, iron 38%, zinc 10%, copper 34%, manganese 66%

HEALTH BENEFITS
Immune system booster | stimulates digestion and circulation

Pear and Pink Peppercorn Smoothie

Preparation time: 5 minutes | Calories per serving: 262

Serves 1

1 pear, peeled, cored and chopped

½ avocado, peeled, pitted and chopped

3 tbsp apple juice

100ml/3½fl oz/scant ½ cup soy milk

3 tbsp plain soy yogurt

2 tsp pink peppercorns

Put all the ingredients in a blender and blend until smooth. Serve immediately.

NUTRIENT BALANCE (per portion)
13% protein, 48% fat, 33% carbohydrate, 6% fibre

VITAMINS AND MINERALS (percentage of RDA)
Vitamin A 2%, E 29%, C 19%, B1 13%, B2 30%, B3 6%, B5 3%, B6 20%, folate 14%, potassium 34%, calcium 9%, magnesium 15%, iron 14%, zinc 6%, copper 33%, manganese 43%

HEALTH BENEFITS
Rich in unsaturated fats and antioxidants | good for circulation | boosts energy

High Energy Punch

Horseradish gives a spicy edge to this fresh, slightly bitter juice, which is packed with fibre, antioxidants, vitamins A and C, and calcium.

Preparation time: 5 minutes | Calories per serving: 122

Serves 1

3 carrots

1 orange

1 small handful of cabbage, spring/collard greens or kale leaves

1 tbsp grated horseradish or fresh wasabi

Juice all the ingredients in an electric juicer and serve immediately. Alternatively, chop the carrots, orange flesh and cabbage leaves, put in a blender with the horseradish and blend together with a little water.

Variation: Use a pinch of dried wasabi instead of fresh horseradish or wasabi.

NUTRIENT BALANCE (per portion)
8% protein, 8% fat, 74% carbohydrate, 13% fibre

VITAMINS AND MINERALS (percentage of RDA)
Vitamin A 391%, E 9%, C 100%, B1 22%, B2 4%, B3 4%, B5 10%, B6 21%, folate 24%, potassium 26%, calcium 12%, magnesium 5%, iron 6%, zinc 4%, copper 11%, manganese 13%, selenium 4%

HEALTH BENEFITS
Antioxidant | immune system booster | good for circulation and bones

Fresh Ginger Ale

Preparation and cooking time: 30 minutes, plus standing and cooling | Calories per serving: 215

Serves 2

75g/2½oz root ginger, peeled and finely chopped
2 whole cloves
100g/3½oz/½ cup raw cane sugar
2 tsp lemon juice
ice cubes and sparkling water, to serve

Bring 300ml/10½fl oz/1¼ cups water to the boil in a small saucepan. Add the ginger and cloves, then turn the heat down to low, cover and leave to simmer for 10 minutes. Tip in the sugar and bring back to the boil, stirring continuously until it dissolves. Lower the heat and simmer for a further 5 minutes, or until the liquid has thickened to a syrup. Remove from the heat and leave to infuse and cool. Strain through a sieve/fine-mesh strainer into a jug/pitcher or glasses, discard the spices and add the lemon juice.

Serve with ice cubes and sparkling water.

NUTRIENT BALANCE (per portion)
1% protein, 2% fat, 95% carbohydrate, 2% fibre

VITAMINS AND MINERALS (percentage of RDA)
Vitamin C 4%, B6 4%, potassium 10%, calcium 5%, magnesium 7%, iron 8%, zinc 2%, copper 6%, manganese 4%

HEALTH BENEFITS
Warming stimulant | good for cold hands and feet | may ease nausea

Summer Elderflower and Lemongrass Cordial

Preparation and cooking time: 45 minutes, plus standing and cooling time |
Calories per serving: 102

Makes 1l/35fl oz/4¼ cups
20 clusters of fresh elderflowers, rinsed
4 lemongrass stalks, pale section only, thinly sliced
500g/17oz grated jaggery, grated or 500g/17oz/2½ cups raw cane sugar

Remove any insects from the rinsed elderflower heads and cut off any stalks and leaves. Pound the lemongrass pieces with a pestle and mortar. Put the sugar and 1l/35fl oz/4¼ cups water in a saucepan over a low heat, and heat for 5 minutes, stirring continuously, until the sugar has dissolved. Bring to the boil, then turn the heat down and leave to simmer for 5 minutes until the syrup thickens slightly. Stir in the elderflowers and lemongrass, remove from the heat and leave to stand for 30 minutes.

Strain the syrup through a fine sieve/strainer. Discard the elderflowers and the lemongrass and pour the syrup into a sterilized bottle. Seal and store in the refrigerator for up to 2 weeks. Serve diluted with water or sparkling water and ice cubes.

Variations: Try mixing with sparkling wine or champagne for a festive drink, or dilute with water and freeze in moulds to make ice lollies/popsicles or flavoured ice cubes.

NUTRIENT BALANCE (per portion)
1% protein, 0% fat, 99% carbohydrate, 0% fibre

VITAMINS AND MINERALS (percentage of RDA)
potassium 6%, calcium 4%, magnesium 11%, iron 5%, copper 25%, manganese 15%

HEALTH BENEFITS
Induces sweating | helps treat colds, sore throats and infections | immune system booster | improves circulation | lowers blood cholesterol

Gløgg (Nordic Mulled Wine)

A traditional Scandinavian hot drink served during the cold, dark winter months.

Preparation and cooking time: 35 minutes, plus standing | Calories per 100ml/ 3½fl oz/scant ½ cup: 228

Serves 6

3–4 tbsp sugar

1 cinnamon stick

3 whole cloves

2.5cm/1in piece of root ginger, peeled and chopped

1 cardamom pod

1 star anise

a pinch of freshly grated nutmeg

150ml/5fl oz/scant ⅔ cup red wine, plus 750ml/26fl oz/3¼ cups red wine or 1l/35fl oz/4¼ cups red grape juice

1 unwaxed orange, sliced

1 unwaxed lemon, sliced

75g/2¼oz/½ cup raisins

50g/1¾oz almonds, skinned and chopped

1 tbsp sugar or honey, or to taste

Put the sugar and spices in a saucepan with 100ml/3½fl oz/scant ½ cup water and the smaller measure of wine. Bring to the boil, turn the heat to low and leave to simmer for 10 minutes. Remove from the heat and leave to infuse for at least 30 minutes.

Strain the liquid into another saucepan and pour in the remaining wine. Add the orange and lemon slices, raisins and almonds. Heat through gently, without boiling, for about 10 minutes. Add honey to taste and serve hot.

NUTRIENT BALANCE (per portion)
6% protein, 21% fat, 70% carbohydrate (incl alcohol), 3% fibre

VITAMINS AND MINERALS (percentage of RDA)
Vitamin E 17%, C 15%, B1 5%, B2 8%, B3 4%, B5 3%, B6 7%, folate 6%, potassium 20%, calcium 10%, magnesium 13%, iron 24%, zinc 6%, copper 24%, manganese 27%

HEALTH BENEFITS
Warming | good for blood and circulation

Spicy Liqueur

Liqueurs are popular in cocktails and as soothing after-dinner digestives, and they are easy and inexpensive to make at home.

Preparation and cooking time: 20 minutes, plus cooling | Maturing time: minimum 2 weeks | Calories per 100ml/3½fl oz/scant ½ cup: 161

Makes 1l/35fl oz/4¼ cups

1 whole clove	6 green cardamom pods
1 tsp allspice	1 cinnamon stick
½ tsp mace	400g/14o/2 cups brown sugar
3 tsp aniseeds	750ml/26fl oz/3¼ cups vodka

Put the spices in a large sealable jar or bottle. Add half the sugar and the vodka, seal the jar and store in the dark for 2 weeks.

Strain the resulting liquid through a muslin cloth/cheesecloth and leave to one side. Boil 100ml/3½fl oz/scant ½ cup water in a saucepan, add the remaining sugar and continue to boil, stirring continuously, until the sugar has dissolved to form a clear syrup. Remove from the heat and leave to cool, then stir in the strained, spiced vodka. Pour into a clean, sterilized bottle and serve immediately. Alternatively, for more intense flavour, leave the liqueur to mature for at least 3 months.

Variations: Use rum or brandy instead of vodka and experiment with different spice combinations.

NUTRIENT BALANCE (per portion)
1% protein, 2% fat, 96% carbohydrate, 1% fibre

VITAMINS AND MINERALS (percentage of RDA)
Potassium 5%, calcium 5%, magnesium 3%, iron 14%, zinc 2%, copper 6%, manganese 6%

HEALTH BENEFITS
Antioxidant | calms digestion | helps to relieve cramps and wind | soothes coughs

GLOSSARY

alkaloids – a group of bitter-tasting, natural chemical compounds. Some are toxic, but many have powerful medicinal actions.

allicin – an organosulfur compound with antibacterial and antifungal properties and a pungent smell. Allicin is found in garlic.

anethole – a volatile oil with oestrogenic properties and a liquorice flavour. It is found in aniseed, fennel and star anise.

annual – a plant that only survives for one growing season.

anthocyanins – red, purple and blue pigments with powerful antioxidant and anti-inflammatory properties.

antibiotic – a treatment for infectious disease that works by killing, or inhibiting the growth of, infecting organisms.

anticoagulant – reduces the tendency of the blood to clot.

antioxidants – chemicals that protect cells from damage caused by unstable molecules known as free radicals.

arbutin – an antimicrobial and mildly diuretic glycoside (see page 230–1).

beta-carotene – a red-orange, fat-soluble antioxidant plant pigment and non-toxic source of vitamin A.

biennial – a plant that blooms in its second year, sets seed and then dies.

bioflavonoids – see flavonoids.

bitter principles – bitter-tasting herbal compounds with a detoxifying action and often used to treat liver complaints.

camphor – a strongly aromatic terpenoid used in food and medicine for its scent and as a local anaesthetic and antimicrobial.

carotenoids – a large group of antioxidant organic pigments, ranging in colour from pale yellow to deep red. They are made during photosynthesis by plants, algae, fungi and some bacteria.

chlorophyll – the light-sensitive green pigment in plants and algae responsible for the synthesis of carbohydrate. It can be used therapeutically for detoxification, and to promote wound healing.

coumarins – sweet-scented phytochemicals that transform into strong anticoagulants in the presence of fungi. They can be used as antiviral, antiseptic, anti-inflammatory, anti-asthmathic, anti-cancer and painkilling remedies.

curcumin – a brightly yellow anti-inflammatory phenol, with potential beneficial effects against many chronic diseases, including cancer. Curcumin is found in turmeric.

deciduous – the botanical term for perennial plants, especially trees and shrubs, that drop their leaves in the autumn.

decoction – a medicinal preparation made by boiling plant material in water (usually for 10–15 minutes) to extract the active ingredients.

diuretic – increases the flow of urine.

ellagic acid – a natural phenolic antioxidant produced by many plants, including pomegranates, that helps protect body cells from oxidative stress.

ellagitannins – antioxidant tannins that may have antibiotic, anti-parasitic and anti-cancer properties. They may help regulate blood glucose levels.

erucic acid – a monounsaturated omega-9 fatty acid of vegetable origin that may protect against cardiovascular disease. It has been found toxic to rats, but no adverse reactions have been documented in humans.

eugenol – an antioxidant and antimicrobial chemical with antiseptic and local anaesthetic properties.

fixed oil – a non-volatile oil, also called a fatty oil.

flavonoids/flavonols – organic plant compounds, sometimes called bioflavonoids or vitamin P, with powerful antioxidant actions. Examples include lutein, zeaxanthin, catechins, betulinic acid, lycopene and xanthines.

free radicals – atoms, molecules or ions that have an uneven number of electrons and which are thus unstable and highly reactive. This reactivity can cause cell damage if there are too many free radicals present in the tissues, and has the potential to cause serious health problems. Antioxidants are important as they neutralize or 'mop up' excess free radicals in the body.

gallic acid – a phenolic acid found in many plants (often forming a part of tannin molecules). It is an antioxidant that has marked antibiotic and astringent properties.

garcinol – a potent antioxidant, anti-cancer and antiviral agent.

glucoside – a glycoside derived from glucose, commonly found in plants.

glycoside – plants often store important phytochemicals in the form of glycosides.

A glycoside molecule consists of sugar bound to another functional substance, for example, alcohol, anthraquinone, coumarin, saponin or a flavonoid, and it is usually these functional molecules that give plants their medicinal effects.

herbaceous – a plant with leaves and stems that die down at the end of the growing season.

hydrogen cyanide – also known as prussic acid, hydrogen cyanide is a highly poisonous chemical found in small amounts in bitter almonds.

kaempferol – a natural flavonoid found in many plants. It has antioxidant, anti-inflammatory, antibiotic and anti-allergic properties, and is associated with a reduced risk of cancer and heart disease.

LDL – sometimes referred to as bad cholesterol, LDL (low-density lipoprotein) is one of a group of lipoproteins that the body uses to transport fats around the circulatory system. High blood levels of LDL are associated with cardiovascular problems.

lignans – a group of antioxidant phytochemicals that includes various phyto-estrogens.

linoleic acid – an unsaturated omega-6 fatty acid. Nigella and poppy seeds contain linoleic acid.

lutein – a yellow to orange-red carotenoid found in plants, egg yolks and animal fats. It is strongly antioxidant, and may protect the eyes from damage resulting from oxidative stress.

lycopene – a bright red carotenoid. Considered a powerful antioxidant, it is also thought to have potential as an anti-cancer agent. Lycopene is also used as a food colouring (E160d).

mucilage – a thick, sticky substance produced by plants that can be used to sooth irritation and inflammation of the skin and mucous membranes.

oleic acid – a naturally occurring monounsaturated omega-9 fatty acid found in olive oil, and in many other vegetable oils and animal fats.

omega oils, 3 and 6 – omega oils are known as essential fatty acids because they are vital to normal health, but can only be obtained from the diet. Omega-3 oils may help relieve cardiovascular problems such as high blood pressure and varicose veins, but in excess they may increase the risk of bleeding and stroke. They are also thought to reduce the severity of symptoms in ADHD and other autistic spectrum disorders in children, and may enhance mental performance in people of all ages. Omega-6 oils are important for normal hormone and prostaglandin production, but the typical Western diet often contains too much omega-6 in relation to omega-3, which can lead to inflammation-related health problems.

oxidative stress – when there are too many free radicals (and other oxidants such as peroxides) in relation to the amount of antioxidants present in the tissues, there is said to be 'oxidative stress'. In this situation, the ability of cells to repair the damage to proteins, fats and DNA is impaired. Oxidative stress is thought to be implicated in many serious chronic health problems, including cancer and cardiovascular problems.

pectin – a polysaccharide found in plant cell walls that can be used as a gelling agent. As pectin is a soluble fibre, eating it as part of a plant-rich diet can help reduce blood cholesterol levels.

perennial – a plant that lives for more than two years.

phenols and polyphenols – a group of organic compounds including tannins, pigments and phyt-hormones that have antioxidant properties.

phytic acid – a chemical found mainly in seeds and grains that is used as an antioxidant, as a food preservative (E391), and in chelation therapy (to treat toxic metal poisoning). It is indigestible for humans but decreases in concentration when seeds and grains are soaked, sprouted or cooked.

phytochemicals – natural compounds in plants that, though not nutrients as such, have a specific biological significance. There are thousands of different phytochemicals in fruit and vegetables with a wide variety of metabolic and medicinal effects. 'Phyto' means 'relating to plants'.

phytoestrogens – plant-derived oestrogens.

phytosterols – plant-derived steroidal compounds similar to cholesterol, found particularly in plant oils. Phytosterols have been shown to lower blood cholesterol and can help maintain normal hormone balance.

pigment – pigments are primarily used by plants for photosynthesis, but also give colour. Examples include chlorophyll, carotenoids, anthocyanins and betalains.

polyphenols – see phenols.

quercetin – an antioxidant bioflavonoid with antihistamine, anti-cancer and anti-inflammatory properties.

RDA – the Recommended Daily Allowance of vitamins, minerals and trace elements considered sufficient to maintain good health. It was developed during the Second World War as part of a broad attempt to improve the nutritional health of the population. RDAs are subect to review and change.

resveratrol – a natural phenol produced by plants to help protect them from natural pathogens. Studies suggest that resveratrol can improve stamina, prevent certain cancers, protect against heart and skin diseases, and act as an anti-diabetic, anti-inflammatory and antiviral.

rhizome – an underground stem used for storing nutrients. Galangal, ginger, turmeric and zedoary are all rhizomes.

salicylic acid/salycilate – a phenolic phytohormone, originally obtained from willow bark (*salix*). It can be used to ease aches and pains, reduce fevers and inflammations and as an antiseptic and food preservative. It also has an anti-diabetic effect. Aspirin is made by reacting salicyclic acid with acetic anhydride in the presence of an acid catalyst.

seitan – is made from wheat gluten and has the texture of cooked meat. It is high in protein, low in fat and carbohydrate, and rich in iron.

shikimic acid – used in the production of antiviral and antibiotic medicines.

tannin – an astringent, tart and bitter polyphenol, used by plants for growth regulation and as a pesticide. Tannin concentrations fall as plants ripen, and they can be used in plant medicine for their astringent, antiviral, antibacterial and anti-parasitic properties.

tempeh – a traditional Indonesian soy product made by fermenting whole soybeans and then pressing them into a firm cake. It has an earthy flavour, and is an extremely good source of protein, fibre and vitamins.

tofu – tofu is made by coagulating soy milk and pressing the curd into solid blocks. There are many different types, but all are low in calories and high in protein.

volatile oil/essential oil – oils that contain volatile aroma compounds that evaporate quickly. Volatile oils often have antiseptic properties.

zeaxanthin – a common carotenoid pigment that gives colour to paprika and many other plants. Diet-derived zeaxanthins contribute one of the main carotenoid pigments in the retina of the eye.

INDEX

ACKNOWLEDGEMENTS

Interesting book and web resources consulted during the writing of this book include:

The NutriCalc database

INTERNET

Wikipedia: en.wikipedia.org

Southwest School of Botanical Medicine:
  swsbm.com

The American Botanical Council:
  abc.herbalgram.org

Harvard Health Publications:
  health.harvard.edu

Self Nutrition Data: nutritiondata.self.com

The Epicentre: theepicentre.com

Spice Advice: spiceadvice.com

MediHerb: mediherb.com

Plants for a Future: pfaf.org

Kew Gardens: kew.org

Royal Horticultural Society: rhs.org.uk

BOOKS

Bartram's Encyclopedia of Herbal Medicine, Thomas Bartram, Robinson Publishing, London 1998

Black Cumin, Peter Schleicher and Mohamed Saleh, Healing Arts Press, Rochester Vermont 2000

Eastern Vegetarian Cooking, Madhur Jaffrey, Arrow Books Ltd, London 1981

Healing Spices, Bharat B. Aggarwal, Sterling Publishing Co, New York 2011

Human Nutrition and Dietetics, 10e; J.S. Garrow, Churchill Livingstone, London 1999

Larousse Gastronomique, Octopus Publishing Group, London 2001

Mighty Spice, John Gregory-Smith, Duncan Baird Publishers Ltd, London 2011

RHS Wisley Experts Gardeners' Advice, The Royal Horticultural Society and Alan R. Toogood, Dorling Kindersley, London 2004

Petit Larousse des Plantes qui Guérissent, Gérard Debuigne and François Couplan, Larousse, Paris 2006

Self-Sufficiency Herbs and Spices, Linda Gray, New Holland Publishers Ltd, London 2011

Slow Cooking Curry and Spice Dishes, Carolyn Humphries, Foulsham, Slough 2011

Spice Spa, Susannah Marriott, Carroll & Brown Publishers Ltd, London 2003

The Oxford Book of Health Foods, J.G. Vaughan and P.A. Judd, Oxford University Press, Oxford 2003

The New Oxford Book of Food Plants, J.G. Vaughan and C.A. Geissler, Oxford University Press, Oxford 1999

The Complete Cook's Encyclopedia of Spices, Sallie Morris and Lesley Mackley, Anness Publishing Ltd, Wigston 2011

The Composition of Foods, McCance and Widdowson, Royal Society of Chemistry, Cambridge, and the Food Standards Agency, London 2002

The Neighborhood Forager, Robert K. Henderson, Chelsea Green Publishing Company, Vermont 2000

The Spice Routes, Chris and Carolyn Caldicott, Frances Lincoln Ltd, London 2001

Food as Medicine, Dharma Singh Khalsa, Atria Books, New York 2003

The Essential Book of Herbal Medicine, Simon Y. Mills, Arkana, London 1993

Caribbean Food Made Easy, Levi Roots, Mitchell Beazley, London 2009

Curry Easy [kindle edition], Madhur Jaffrey, Ebury Digital 2011

Indian Vegetarian Feast, Anjum Anand, Sterling Epicure, New York 2013

THE AUTHOR WOULD LIKE TO THANK

Allan Hartvig	Essie Jain	Peter Firebrace
Ann Britt Fogde	Jennifer Maughan	Raphael Charmetant
Anna Mews	Kirsten Hansen	Ric Wilkinson
Carolyn Ryden	Linda Wilkinson	Rob Ward
Catherine Argence	Lonnie Nielsen	Robert Saxton
Cecile Charmetant	Maya Morgan	Roger Walton
Charlotte Charmetant	Michaela Morgan	Steen Piper
Charlotte Yde	Nic Rowley	Tessa Hodsdon
Emilie Rose	Paul Charmetant	Yann Jautard

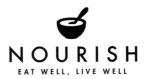

NOURISH
EAT WELL, LIVE WELL

Here at Nourish we're all about wellbeing through food and drink – irresistible dishes with a serious good-for-you factor. If you want to eat and drink delicious things that set you up for the day, suit any special diets, keep you healthy and make the most of the ingredients you have, we've got some great ideas to share with you. Come over to our blog for wholesome recipes and fresh inspiration – **nourishbooks.com**.